RNC-OB® EXAM PREP STUDY GUIDE

RNC-OB® EXAM PREP STUDY GUIDE

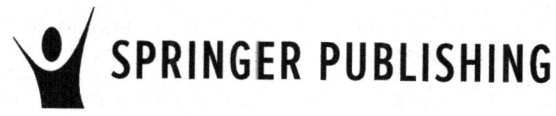

Copyright © 2024 Springer Publishing Company, LLC
All rights reserved.

No part of this publication may be reproduced, stored in a retrieval system, or transmitted in any form or by any means, electronic, mechanical, photocopying, recording, or otherwise, without the prior permission of Springer Publishing Company, LLC, or authorization through payment of the appropriate fees to the Copyright Clearance Center, Inc., 222 Rosewood Drive, Danvers, MA 01923, 978-750-8400, fax 978-646-8600, info@copyright.com or at www.copyright.com.

Springer Publishing Company, LLC
11 West 42nd Street, New York, NY 10036
www.springerpub.com

Acquisitions Editor: Jaclyn Koshofer
Content Development Editor: Julia Curcio
Compositor: Exeter Premedia Services Private Ltd.

ISBN: 978-0-8261-6579-4
ebook ISBN: 978-0-8261-6629-6
DOI: 10.1891/ 9780826166296

23 24 25 26 / 5 4 3 2 1

The author and the publisher of this Work have made every effort to use sources believed to be reliable to provide information that is accurate and compatible with the standards generally accepted at the time of publication. The author and publisher shall not be liable for any special, consequential, or exemplary damages resulting, in whole or in part, from the readers' use of, or reliance on, the information contained in this book. The publisher has no responsibility for the persistence or accuracy of URLs for external or third-party Internet websites referred to in this publication and does not guarantee that any content on such websites is, or will remain, accurate or appropriate.

RNC-OB® is a registered trademark of National Certification Corporation (NCC). NCC does not endorse this resource, nor does it have a proprietary relationship with Springer Publishing Company.

Library of Congress Control Number: 2022952381

Contact sales@springerpub.com to receive discount rates on bulk purchases.

Publisher's Note: **New and used products purchased from third-party sellers are not guaranteed for quality, authenticity, or access to any included digital components.**

Printed in the United States of America by Gasch Printing.

CONTENTS

Preface ix
Pass Guarantee xi

1. GENERAL EXAMINATION INFORMATION 1

Overview 1
Certification Requirements 1
About the Examination 1
Five Categories of Question Topics 1
Scoring 2
How to Apply 2
How to Recertify 2
NCC Contact Information 3

2. COMPLICATIONS OF PREGNANCY 5

Rh Incompatibility 5
Immune System 5
Antiphospholipid Syndrome 5
Systematic Lupus Erythematosus 6
Rheumatoid Arthritis 7
Scleroderma 8
Cardiovascular System 9
Congenital Heart Defects 9
Heart Valve Defects 10
Rhythm Disorders 11
Hypertensive Disorders 12
Pregestational/Chronic Hypertension 12
Gestational Hypertension 12
HELLP Syndrome 13
Eclampsia 14
Severe Hypertension/Hypertension Emergency 15
Endocrine Disorders 16
Diabetes Mellitus 16
Type 1 Diabetes 18
Type 2 Diabetes 19
Hypothyroidism 20
Hyperthyroidism 21
Gastrointestinal System 22
Cholelithiasis 22
Cholestasis 23
Fatty Liver 24
Obesity 25
Pregnancy After Bariatric Surgery 25
Hematopoetic Anemia 26
Disseminated Intravascular Coagulation 27
Hemolytic Disease 28
Thrombocytopenia 29
Thrombophilia 30
Infectious Disease Bacterial Vaginosis 31
COVID-19 32
Chlamydia 32
Gonorrhea 33
Group Beta Strep 34
Herpes 34
HIV Infection 35
Human Papillomavirus 36
Influenza 37

Zika Virus   37
Syphilis   38
Urinary Tract Infection   39
Multiple Gestation   40
**Amniotic Fluid Assessment
   Oligohydramnios**   41
Polyhydramnios   42
Appendix 2.1: Medications for DM in Pregnancy   43
Resources   44

3. FETAL ASSESSMENT   49

Antenatal Testing   49
Amniocentesis   49
Contraction Stress Test   50
Fetal Growth Evaluation   51
Nonstress Test   51
Percutaneous Umbilical Cord Blood Sampling   52
Quad Screen Test   53
Biophysical Profile   53
Umbilical Artery Doppler Flow Studies   54
Glucose Tolerance Test   54
Fetal Monitoring   55
Fetal Heart Rate Assessment   55
Electronic Fetal Monitoring   55
Dysrhythmias   56
Tachycardia   56
Bradycardia   56
Variability   57
Artifact   58
Accelerations and Decelerations   58
Fetal Heart Rate Categories   62
Fetal Scalp Electrode   64
Uterine Activity Assessment   64
Intrauterine Resuscitation   66
Resources   67

4. LABOR AND BIRTH   69

Physiology   69
Maternal Physiology   69
Physical Assessment   69
General Assessment   69
Abdominal Assessment   70
Vaginal Assessment   71
Stages of Labor   71
Induction of Labor: Considerations   73
Indications   73
Contraindications   73
Complications   74
Bishop Score   74
Induction of Labor: Methods   74
Cook Balloon and Foley Catheter   74
Amniotomy   74
Mechanical Methods   75
Oxytocin Infusion   75
Prostaglandins   76
Pain Management and Coping   76
Nonpharmacologic Methods   76
Birthing and Peanut Balls   76
Coaching   76
Hydrotherapy   77
Positioning   77
Relaxation and Guided Imagery   77
Pharmacologic Methods   77
Narcotics   77
Nitrous Oxide   78
Regional Anesthesia   78
General Anesthesia   79
Labor Procedures   80
Cesarean Birth   80
Vaginal Birth After Cesarean   81
Episiotomy   81
Operative Vaginal Delivery   82

Labor Complications 83	Postpartum Depression 100
Prolonged Pregnancy 83	Postpartum Psychosis 100
Breech or Transverse Presentation 83	**The Newborn** 101
Shoulder Dystocia 84	Neonatal Resuscitation 101
Amniotic Fluid Embolism 85	Adaptation to Extrauterine Life 102
Prolapsed Umbilical Cord 85	Initial Newborn Assessment 103
Premature Rupture of Membranes 86	**Body Systems Assessment of the Newborn** 104
Prolonged Rupture of Membranes 86	Skin 104
Chorioamnionitis 87	Head and Neck 105
Appendix 4.1: Medications for Induction of Labor 87	Mouth 106
Appendix 4.2: Medications for Pain During Labor 88	Eyes and Nose 107
Resources 88	Limbs 107

5. RECOVERY, POSTPARTUM, AND NEWBORN CARE 91

Postpartum 91	Chest and Cardiovascular 108
Postpartum Assessments 91	Abdomen 108
Perineum 91	Genitalia/Anus 109
Fundal Height 92	Back/Spine/Hips 109
Lochia 92	Neurologic 110
Pain Assessment 92	Behavior States 110
Incision Assessment 93	**Newborn Complications** 111
Wound Vacuum 93	Late Preterm Infants 111
Recovery/Postpartum Complications 93	Brachial Plexus Injury 113
Overview 93	Laceration 114
Cardiomyopathy 94	Hypoglycemia 114
Hematoma 94	Jaundice 115
Laceration 95	Newborn Infections 116
Infections 95	Neonatal Abstinence Syndrome 117
Retained Products 96	**Laboratory Evaluation** 118
Thromboembolic Deep Vein Thrombosis 97	Rh Incompatibility 118
Postpartum Hemorrhage 98	Anemia 119
Mental Health 99	Polycythemia 120
Overview 99	Thrombocytopenia 121
Postpartum Anxiety 100	**Infant Nutrition** 122
	Breastfeeding 122
	Breastfeeding Complications 123
	Mastitis 123

Inability to Latch 123
Formula Feeding 124
Safe Handling 124
Bottle Feeding Technique 124
Inhibiting Milk Production 124
Parent–Infant Bonding 124
Rooming-In 125
Skin-To-Skin Contact 125
Signs of Inadequate Bonding 125
Perinatal Loss and Grief 125
Recommendations After Discharge 125
Newborn Care and Safety 125
Common Newborn Concerns 126
Postpartum Patient Care 127
Appendix 5.1: Medications for Postpartum Complications 128
Resources 129

6. **PROFESSIONAL PRACTICE** 131
Professional Issues 131
Ethics 131
Legal Issues 132
Evidence-Based Practice and Quality Improvement 133
Perinatal Core Measures 133
Quality and Performance Improvement 134
Overview 134
Postpartum Hemorrhage 135
Induction Protocols 136
Timely Management of Severe Hypertension 136
Decreasing Racial Disparity 136
Postpartum Warning Signs 136
Research Terminology 137
Resources 138

7. **PRACTICE TEST QUESTIONS** 141
8. **PRACTICE TEST ANSWERS** 173
9. **ANSWERS TO POP QUIZ QUESTIONS** 205

Index 207
Abbreviations Inside back cover

PREFACE

This *Exam Prep Study Guide* was designed to be a high-speed review—a last-minute gut check before your exam day. We created this review to supplement to your certification preparation studies. We encourage you to use it in conjunction with other study aids to ensure you are as prepared as possible for the exam.

This book follows National Certification Corporation's most recent exam content outlines and uses a succinct, bulleted format to highlight what you need to know. The aim of this book is to help you solidify your retention of information in the month or so leading up to your exam. It is written by certified inpatient obstetric nurses who are familiar with the exam and the content you need to know Special features appear throughout the book to call out important information, including:

- **Complications**: Problems that can arise with certain disease states or procedures
- **Nursing Pearls**: Additional patient care insights and strategies for knowledge retention
- **Alerts**: Need-to-know details on how to handle emergency situations or when to transfer care
- **Pop Quizzes**: Critical-thinking questions to test your ability to synthesize what you learned (answers in the back of the book)
- **Two Full-Length Practice Tests**: One printed in the book, one online
- **Free One-Month Access to ExamPrepConnect**: The digital study platform that guides you confidently through your exam prep journey

We know life is busy. Being able to prepare for your exam efficiently and effectively is paramount, which is why we created this *Exam Prep Study Guide*. You have come to the right place as you continue on your path of professional growth and development. The stakes are high, and we want to help you succeed. Best of luck to you on your certification journey. You've got this!

PASS GUARANTEE

If you use this resource to prepare for your exam and do not pass, you may return it for a refund of your full purchase price, excluding tax, shipping, and handling. To receive a refund, return your product along with a copy of your exam score report and original receipt showing purchase of new product (not used). Product must be returned and received within 180 days of the original purchase date. Refunds will be issued within 8 weeks from acceptance and approval. One offer per person and address. This offer is valid for U.S. residents only. Void where prohibited. To initiate a refund, please contact Customer Service at csexamprep@springerpub.com.

1 GENERAL EXAMINATION INFORMATION

OVERVIEW

- The National Certification Corporation (NCC), founded in 1975 as a not-for-profit organization, offers multiple core certifications and specialty certifications. These certifications are accredited by the National Commission for Certifying Agencies.
- The RNC-OB® examination is a competency-based exam that assesses knowledge of nursing care of the inpatient obstetric patient and the application of that knowledge. It is intended for registered nurses in both the United States and Canada who take care of patients during the antepartum, intrapartum, and postpartum periods.
- The NCC is not a licensure organization. Certain standards regarding practice and education requirements are in place to qualify for the exam, but the certification has no bearing on individual licensing to practice.

CERTIFICATION REQUIREMENTS

To be eligible to sit for the RNC-OB® exam, test takers must meet the following requirements:
- Have a current, unencumbered nursing license in either the United States or Canada.
- Have a minimum of 2 years of experience caring for the hospitalized patient in the antepartum, intrapartum, postpartum, and neonatal periods.

ABOUT THE EXAMINATION

- The RNC-OB® examination is a 3-hour exam with up to 175 questions.
- Of the 175 test questions, 150 are scored, and the rest are embedded as pretest questions.
- The focus of the exam is on pregnant patients after 20 weeks of gestation through postpartum discharge.
- Each question is multiple choice with a full premise and three possible answers. All questions are designed the same, and each answer group is organized in alphabetical order.
- The exam is computerized, and each test is administered in random order for different candidates.
- Questions are designed to assess knowledge and the application of knowledge. They are broken down into five categories.

FIVE CATEGORIES OF QUESTION TOPICS

- **Complications of pregnancy (29%):** Maternal complications affecting the fetus and newborn, maternal psychological and environmental factors, preterm labor, multiple gestation, and placental disorders
- **Fetal assessment (18%):** Antenatal testing, electronic fetal monitoring, non-electronic fetal monitoring, acid–base interpretation ▶

FIVE CATEGORIES OF QUESTION TOPICS (*continued*)

- **Labor and birth (35%):** Physiology of labor, assessment and management of labor, obstetric and perioperative procedures, pain management and coping, labor and obstetric complications, induction, and augmentation
- **Recovery, postpartum, and newborn care (15%):** Recovery and postpartum physiology and complications, family dynamics and discharge readiness, lactation and infant nutrition, newborn physiology, and complications
- **Professional issues (3%):** Legal, ethics, safety, and quality improvement

SCORING

- Scoring for the exam is pass/fail.
- A passing score is based on a predetermined set of criteria established by the Content Team.
- These criteria are based on the evaluation of clinical significance of content and the past statistical performance of test questions.
- Questions used to determine pass/fail have been statistically proven to be an appropriate measure of an individual's ability and knowledge.
- There is no set percentage score for a passing level.
- The passing of each candidate is based on the number of questions they answer correctly, and there is no penalty for wrong answers.
- Pass/fail is determined based on ability level using the process of equating. This determination means that someone who takes a slightly more difficult exam will need to answer fewer questions correctly to pass than will a candidate who receives a slightly less difficult exam.
- Test reports indicate a pass/fail status and feedback on strengths and weaknesses in the content areas tested.

HOW TO APPLY

- Applications for the exam are accepted online only on the NCC website. NCC sends confirmation via email if applicants are approved.
- Once approved, applicants have 90 days from the date of the application to take the exam and must schedule it within the first 30 days of the eligibility window.
- The exam cost is $325, including a nonrefundable $50 application fee.
- If unable to keep the original date, a change request may be made for an additional fee of $125.
- Additional fees may be incurred for changing the exam category, withdrawing from the exam, and submitting incomplete applications. Details can be found on the NCC website at NCCwebsite.org.
- Candidates who are unsuccessful may retake the exam. They must reapply and pay all applicable fees. The retest application must be completed no sooner than 90 days after the date of the original exam.

HOW TO RECERTIFY

- After successfully passing the RNC-OB® examination, certification is active for 3 years.
- Nurses who want to maintain certification must obtain specific hours of continuing education (CE) credit as defined in the Education Plan, which is determined by their Continuing Competency Assessment (CCA).
- Nurses may apply for recertification up to 1 year before their expiration date, as long as they have completed the CE requirements. ▶

HOW TO RECERTIFY (*continued*)

- CE requirements must be obtained after the CCA is completed to be eligible.
- Recertification is due in the quarter in which the passing notification was originally received. This due date is listed on the applicant's account on the NCC website.

NCC CONTACT INFORMATION

Details of the exam are subject to change. For the most up-to-date information, please contact the NCC:
National Certification Corporation
676 N. Michigan Avenue, Suite 3600
Chicago, IL 60611
Website: www.NCCwebsite.org
Email: info@nccnet.org

For information on recertification, visit https://www.NCCwebsite.ort/content/documents/cms/cca-steps.pdf
For CCA examples, visit: https://www.NCCwebsite.org/content/documents/cms/cca-education-plans.pdf

2 COMPLICATIONS OF PREGNANCY

RH INCOMPATIBILITY
Overview

- Rh incompatibility occurs when there is mixing of maternal Rh-negative blood and fetal Rh-positive blood during pregnancy, causing the pregnant patient to produce Rh-positive antibodies. Production of Rh-positive antibodies is more likely to occur in subsequent pregnancies rather than in the first pregnancy. Rh incompatibility affects the fetus because maternal blood recognizes the fetal blood as a foreign substance. Rh incompatibility may cause serious health problems or even death to the fetus or newborn.
- Rho(D) immune globulin (RhoGAM) is administered to Rh-negative unsensitized (without Rh-positive antibodies) patients at 28 weeks' gestation to protect the fetus from red blood cell destruction. RhoGAM provides maternal passive antibodies so that maternal blood does **not** recognize fetal Rh-positive blood as a foreign substance. Rh-negative postpartum patients should receive a dose of RhoGAM within 72 hours of infant delivery.

[ ] **COMPLICATIONS**

All unsensitized Rh-negative patients who have had an abortion, ectopic pregnancy, chorionic villous sampling, amniocentesis, or birth of an Rh-positive infant should receive RhoGAM to prevent Rh-positive antibodies from developing.

IMMUNE SYSTEM
ANTIPHOSPHOLIPID SYNDROME
Overview

- Antiphospholipid syndrome (APS) is an autoimmune disorder in which there is a production of antiphospholipid antibodies. This disease often occurs in the presence of systemic lupus erythematosus (SLE).

Signs and Symptoms

- **Frequent blood clots**: Blood clot symptoms depend on where the blood clot occurs in the body and include chest pain and shortness of breath; pain, redness, or swelling in arms or legs; recurrent headaches, seizures, or migraines; stroke; and abdominal pain.
- **Complications of pregnancy**: Complications include recurrent pregnancy loss, preeclampsia, preterm deliveries; mottled, blue, netlike pattern on skin.

Diagnosis

- **Vascular thrombosis**: Venous, arterial, or small vessel thrombosis in any tissue or organ; imaging and blood studies support evidence of thrombosis
- **Pregnancy loss**: One or more unexplained losses of a normal pregnancy of ≥10 weeks' gestation; premature births of <34 weeks' gestation due to preeclampsia, eclampsia, or placental insufficiency; or three or more unexplained spontaneous pregnancy losses at <10 weeks

Labs
- Anticardiolipin (aCL) antibodies (IgG and IgM)
- Anti-beta2-glycoprotein 1
- Lupus anticoagulant

Diagnostic Testing
- Ultrasound of extremities

Treatment
- **Antiplatelet agent**: low-dose aspirin
- **Anticoagulants**: enoxaparin or heparin

Nursing Interventions
- Assess blood pressure (BP), IV sites, capillary refill, and level of consciousness regularly.
- Monitor urinary output hourly.
- Monitor for venous and arterial blood clots.

Patient Education
- Take medication as prescribed.
- **Monitor for signs of bleeding**: Watch for unexplained bleeding from gums or nose, bright red or coffee-ground vomit, or blood in stool or tarlike appearance of stool.
- **Monitor for signs of stroke**: Watch for sudden weakness on one side of body, slurred speech or sudden confusion, and trouble seeing or walking.
- **Manage risk factors for developing clots**: Control diabetes, hypertension, and cholesterol; stop smoking.

SYSTEMATIC LUPUS ERYTHEMATOSUS (SLE)

Overview
- SLE is a chronic, inflammatory, multisystem autoimmune disease where the body attacks any organ or system in the body. Patients with SLE are advised to be on pregnancy-safe medications for 6 months without a flare prior to conceiving.
- SLE increases risk of preterm delivery, intrauterine growth restriction (IUGR), and stillbirth.

Signs and Symptoms
- Fatigue
- Fever, temperature of 100°F (37.8°C)
- Muscle pain or tenderness
- Weight changes (gain or loss)
- Joint pain, stiffness, swelling, or arthritis
- Skin rashes
- Sun sensitivity
- Oral ulcers
- Problems with heart, lungs or kidneys

Diagnosis
Labs
- Complete blood count (CBC)
- Comprehensive metabolic panel (CMP) ▶

Labs (continued)
- Creatinine
- Urinalysis
- Antinuclear antibody
- Anti–double-stranded DNA
- Antiphospholipid antibodies
- C-reactive protein
- Uric acid
- Protein to creatinine (PC) ratio

Diagnostic Testing
- Imaging may be valuable, but it is not routinely performed unless indicated by other clinical findings.

Treatment
- Steroids
- **Aspirin**: Protection against preeclampsia

Nursing Interventions
- Assess skin condition and integrity.
- Monitor vital signs and urine output.
- Provide comfort measures.
- Control pain.
- Encourage healthy lifestyle activities.
- Monitor for fetal movement and kick counts.
- Implement preterm labor precautions.

Patient Education
- Take medication as prescribed.
- Eat a well-balanced diet, exercise regularly, and get adequate rest.
- Monitor kick counts starting at 27 weeks.
- Watch for signs and symptoms of preterm labor.
- Notify provider of any changes in health.

RHEUMATOID ARTHRITIS (RA)
Overview
- RA is an autoimmune inflammatory disorder that mostly affects synovial joints but can affect skin, eyes, heart, and blood vessels. Most pregnant patients with RA see an improvement in symptoms during pregnancy. It is typical for postpartum patients to have a flare.

Signs and Symptoms
- Fatigue
- Swelling of hands, feet, or ankles
- Joint pain

Diagnosis
Labs
- Erythrocyte sedimentation rate ▶

Labs (continued)
- C-reactive protein
- Rheumatoid factor
- Anti-cyclic citrullinated peptide (CCP) antibodies

Diagnostic Testing
- X-rays of involved joints

Treatment
- Hydroxychloroquine
- Sulfasalazine
- Tumor necrosis factor alpha inhibitor
- Targeted synthetic disease-modifying antirheumatic drugs

Nursing Interventions
- Provide pain relief.
- Provide comfort measures.
- Maintain functional mobility.
- Monitor for preterm labor.

Patient Education
- Take medications as prescribed.
- Physical therapy may be necessary.
- Monitor fetal movements and kick counts.
- Be watchful for signs of preterm labor.

SCLERODERMA
Overview
- Scleroderma is a rare disease that involves hardening and tightening of skin and connective tissues.

Signs and Symptoms
- Puffy skin that becomes itchy, tight, or thick
- Joint pain and stiffness
- Fatigue
- Intense response to cold
- Fingers and toes turning white or purple-blue
- Heartburn or trouble swallowing
- Poor appetite or weight loss
- Damage to organs

Diagnosis
Labs
- CBC
- Serum creatinine
- Creatine kinase
- Urinalysis with urine sediment
- Antibody tests

Diagnostic Testing
- Imaging on organs affected, pulmonary function test, echocardiography, skin biopsy

Treatment
- Heartburn medication
- Pain medications
- Calcium channel blockers
- Corticosteroids

Nursing Interventions
- Implement pain control.
- Monitor urinary output.
- Monitor fetal well-being.
- Monitor vital signs, especially BP.
- Assess skin, heart, lungs, and kidneys.

Patient Education
- Exercise regularly.
- Drink plenty of fluids.
- Monitor BP.
- Monitor fetal movements and kick counts.
- Report flares or changes in health.

CARDIOVASCULAR SYSTEM

CONGENITAL HEART DEFECTS (CHDS)

Overview
- Due to advances in technology and medicine, people born with CHDs are now reaching reproductive age. The majority of maternal deaths due to cardiovascular issues occur during delivery or in the first week postpartum. CHDs can often cause arrhythmias.

Signs and Symptoms
- Cyanosis
- Tachypnea
- Dyspnea
- Fatigue
- Murmur
- Arrhythmias
- Edema

Diagnosis
Labs
- CBC
- Prothrombin time (PT), partial thromboplastin time (PTT)
- Comprehensive medical panel (CMP)
- Drug screen ▶

Labs (continued)
- Thyroid-stimulating hormone (TSH)
- Artreial blood gas (ABG)

Diagnostic Testing
- Pulse oximetry
- Echocardiogram
- Transesophageal echo
- Cardiac computed tomography (CT) and magnetic resonance imaging (MRI)
- Chest x-ray (CXR)

Treatment
- **Anticoagulation regimen (depending on type):** minimizes thromboembolism
- Surgical repair

Nursing Interventions
- Maintain oxygen saturation at appropriate levels during labor.
- Avoid supine positioning during labor and birth.
- Implement hemodynamic monitoring.
- Perform capillary refill assessment.
- Monitor fetal status for decreased variability or uteroplacental insufficiency.

HEART VALVE DEFECTS

Overview
- During pregnancy there is an increase in heart rate (HR), cardiac output, and stroke volume. These cardiac changes in pregnancy can cause rapid decompensation in patients with heart valve defects. Risks and complications depend on type of heart valve defect.

Signs and Symptoms
- Fatigue
- Shortness of breath
- Finger clubbing
- Murmur
- Lightheadedness and fatigue
- Tachycardia
- Persistent cough
- Increased urination at night
- Swelling of the feet, hands, ankles, and arms

Diagnosis
Labs
- Cardiac biomarkers

Diagnostic Testing
- Cardiac imaging
- Echocardiogram
- Stress test

Treatment

- Surgical treatment during pregnancy not advised
- Anticoagulants

Nursing Interventions

- Closely monitor input and output as valve defects increase the risk for fluid overload.
- Monitor hemodynamic changes, pulse pressure, mean arterial pressure (MAP), and HR changes.
- Administer oxygen based on pulse oximetry findings.
- Use side-lying position with head and shoulders elevated.
- Provide comfort measures such as low light and calm environment.
- Perform capillary refill assessment.
- Monitor for edema.

Patient Education

- Avoid alcohol and smoking.
- Avoid stimulants such as caffeine.
- Report any changes, such as shortness of breath (SOB), productive cough, edema, or lightheadedness.

RHYTHM DISORDERS

Overview

- Arrhythmias are the most common cardiac complication in pregnancy. Patients with existing arrhythmias or congenital heart defects (CHD) are at highest risk for developing an arrhythmia during pregnancy.

COMPLICATIONS

Not treating tachycardia arrhythmias can lead to cardiomyopathy.

Signs and Symptoms

- Palpitations or fluttering in the chest
- Dizziness or lightheadedness
- Tachycardia or bradycardia depending on type of arrhythmia

Diagnosis

Diagnostic Testing
- Electrocardiogram (EKG)

Treatment

- Medications
- Cardioversion
- Implantable cardioverter-defibrillator

Nursing Interventions

- Assess HR and sound.
- Monitor for changes in work of breathing.
- Administer medications as scheduled.
- Monitor fetal well-being.

Patient Education

- Avoid stimulants such as caffeine.
- Avoid alcohol and smoking.
- Report any changes, such as SOB, productive cough, edema, or lightheadedness.

HYPERTENSIVE DISORDERS

PREGESTATIONAL/CHRONIC HYPERTENSION

Overview

- *Chronic hypertension* is defined as BP greater than or equal to 140 mm Hg systolic and/or 90 mmHg diastolic before pregnancy or before 20 weeks of gestation. About 25% of patients with pregestational hypertension will develop preeclampsia.

Signs and Symptoms

- Headaches
- Vision changes (blurry or double vision)
- May be asymptomatic

Diagnosis

Labs
- CBC (baseline)
- Urinalysis (baseline)

Treatment

- The medications most safe to use in pregnancy are labetalol, nifedipine, hydralazine, methyldopa, and low-dose aspirin.

Nursing Interventions

- Monitor vital signs at regular intervals.
- Keep environment calm.
- Monitor fetal well-being.

Patient Education

- Monitor BP at home.
- Report if BP changes are higher than normal.
- Monitor fetal status.

GESTATIONAL HYPERTENSION

Overview

- *Gestational hypertension* is characterized by systolic BP of 140 mm Hg or more or diastolic BP of 90 mmHg or more, or both, on two occasions at least 4 hours apart after 20 weeks' gestation, without the presence of protein in the urine. It often proceeds to preeclampsia.

Signs and Symptoms

- Headaches
- Vision changes (blurry or double vision)

Diagnosis
Labs
- Urinalysis for protein

Treatment
- Medications most safe to use pregnancy are labetalol, nifedipine, and hydralazine.

Nursing Interventions
- Assess for new onset of edema.
- Monitor vital signs at regular intervals.
- Keep environment calm.

Patient Education
- Take medications as prescribed.
- Monitor BP at home.
- Report higher-than-normal BP.
- Monitor fetal movement/well-being.

HELLP SYNDROME
Overview
- Hemolysis, elevated liver enzymes and low platelets (HELLP) syndrome is diagnosed in patients with hemolysis, elevated liver enzymes, and low platelet count. Half of patients affected by HELLP also have preeclampsia.

[ ] **COMPLICATIONS**

With increased intrabdominal pressure, a subscapular hematoma can rupture, causing internal bleeding, hypovolemic shock, and fetal and maternal mortality. Additional complications are maternal bleeding and preterm deliveries.

Signs and Symptoms
- Pain or tenderness in upper right quadrant of abdomen or midepigastric region
- Nausea or vomiting
- Severe edema
- Flu-like symptoms
- Headaches
- Visual changes
- Shoulder pain with deep breaths
- Bleeding
- Shortness of breath
- High BP

Diagnosis
Labs
- CBC
- Liver function
- Creatinine
- Bilirubin

Treatment

- Close observation of maternal and fetal monitoring
- Control of hypertension
- Magnesium sulfate administration
- Immediate delivery
- Low-dose aspirin (ASA)

Nursing Interventions

- Assess pain regularly and provide pain management.
- Assist patient to comfortable position.
- Assess respiratory status frequently.
- Monitor fetal status with continuous fetal monitoring.
- Administer medications per order.

Patient Education

- Report shortness of breath.
- Report changes in status, if worsened.
- Take medications as directed.
- Know that transfer to a tertiary care center may be necessary during labor.

ECLAMPSIA

Overview

- *Preeclampsia* is associated with new-onset hypertension, which occurs most often after 20 weeks' gestation, often near term.
- Preeclampsia is often accompanied by new-onset proteinuria.
- Hypertension and other signs or symptoms of preeclampsia may present in some patients without proteinuria.
- Preeclampsia is often diagnosed with gestational hypertension and proteinuria (greater than or equal to 300 mg in 24-hour collection or a protein/creatinine ratio of greater than or equal to 0.3 mg/dL).
- **Gestational hypertension in the absence of proteinuria is diagnosed with preeclampsia with severe features if any of the following are present**: Impaired liver function, new-onset headache, pulmonary edema, renal insufficiency, severe persistent right upper-quadrant or epigastric pain, systolic BP of 160 mm Hg or higher, diastolic BP of 110 mm Hg or higher, thrombocytopenia (platelet count less than 100,000), visual disturbances.

COMPLICATIONS

Complications for the fetus include fetal growth restriction and preterm birth. Complications to maternal body systems include cardiovascular effects, eclampsia, HELLP syndrome, liver damage, renal damage, retinal damage, placental abruption, pulmonary edema, and neurologic effects such as hypertensive encephalopathy. In addition, stroke is the leading cause of maternal morbidity from preeclampsia.

Signs and Symptoms

- Severe persistent right upper quadrant or epigastric pain
- Visual disturbances
- Sudden weight gain
- Swelling in hands, feet, and face
- Headache unrelieved by acetaminophen
- Hyperreflexia ▶

Signs and Symptoms (*continued*)
- Crackles in lungs
- Decreased urine output

Diagnosis
Labs
- Protein-creatine ratio
- CBC
- aspartate transaminase/alanine transaminase (AST/ALT)

Treatment
- Antihypertensive medications safe in pregnancy include labetalol, nifedipine, and hydralazine.
- Preeclampsia/eclampsia treatment includes magnesium sulfate.
- Seizure treatment includes the anticonvulsants lorazepam, diazepam, phenytoin, and Keppra.

[ ] **NURSING PEARLS**

Treat BP with antihypertensives. To reduce the risk of seizures or to treat eclampsia, use magnesium sulfate.

Nursing Interventions
- Assess daily weight and signs of edema.
- Monitor vital signs closely, specifically BP.
- Monitor input/output (I/O) closely.
- Assess deep tendon reflexes.
- Assess lung sounds for signs of pulmonary edema.
- Assess for headache unrelieved by medication, level of consciousness, neurologic status for magnesium toxicity, and visual changes.
- Assess FHR.
- Use seizure precautions: pad the bed and have suction and yanker ready for use.

Patient Education
- Report headache, lightheadedness, or dizziness.
- Report shortness of breath.
- Report decreased fetal movements.

SEVERE HYPERTENSION/HYPERTENSION EMERGENCY
Overview
- **Severe range BPs, measured at least 4 hours apart, with one of the following**: systolic BP of 160 mmHg or higher or diastolic BP of 110 mmHg or higher
- **Hypertensive emergency**: occurs when two severe BPs are taken 15 to 60 minutes apart; severe values do not need to be consecutive.

Signs and Symptoms
- Severe range blood pressures: two severe BPs >160/110, taken 15 to 60 minutes apart

Diagnosis

Labs
- CBC
- CMP
- Liver enzymes
- blood urea nitrogen (BUN) and creatinine
- Urinalysis

Treatment

- Antihypertensive medications safe in pregnancy: labetalol, nifedipine, and hydralazine
- For prevention of seizures: magnesium sulfate
- For seizure treatment: lorazepam, diazepam, phenytoin, keppra

Nursing Interventions

- Monitor BP closely.
- Monitor fetal status closely.
- Monitor I/O closely.
- Administer medications as ordered.
- Maintain magnesium sulfate infusion.
- Take seizure precautions.

Patient Education

- Take medications as prescribed.
- Know that NICU staff may need to attend delivery.

ENDOCRINE DISORDERS

DIABETES MELLITUS (DM)

Overview

- DM is a disorder of carbohydrate metabolism in which insulin production is greatly reduced or stopped. Without insulin, glucose cannot be carried across the cell membrane. This accumulation of glucose in the blood stream is known as hyperglycemia.
- Two types of diabetes mellitus can occur during pregnancy: gestational and pregestational. *Gestational diabetes mellitus (GDM)* is a condition of carbohydrate intolerance that occurs during pregnancy. It typically occurs and is diagnosed at 24 to 28 weeks' gestation. GDM usually resolves after delivery, although up to one third of patients could still have abnormal glucose testing at their postpartum screening, and 15% to 70% of these patients could develop diabetes later in life. There are two types of GDM: A1GDM (diet-controlled GDM) and A2GDM: GDM requiring medication. *Pregestational diabetes mellitus (pregestational DM)* is a condition affecting 1% to 2% of all pregnant patients. It is a complicated disease that can affect both the patient and the fetus. Type 1 DM is thought to be an autoimmune reaction that destroys the beta cells in the pancreas that make insulin, leading to absolute insulin deficiency. Type 2 DM develops in the presence of an insulin secretory defect. Pancreatic cells do not respond to insulin properly, resulting in the increased work of the pancreas and a rise in blood glucose.

COMPLICATIONS

Pregnant patients with DM are at risk for preeclampsia, hypoglycemia, hyperglycemia, stillbirth, and preterm labor. A fetus of a patient with DM is at risk for birth defects, macrosomia, and polyhydramnios. After birth, the neonate is at risk for hypoglycemia. Diabetic ketoacidosis (DKA) can result if the body doesn't produce enough insulin to break down glucose into energy. Instead, the body breaks down fat, causing the liver to create ketones, which makes the blood acidic and can be fatal if untreated.

Signs and Symptoms

- Signs and symptoms of GDM, pregestational DM, and DKA include blurred vision, dry mouth, fatigue and weakness, polydipsia, polyuria, unexplained weight loss, nausea, and vomiting.

Diagnosis

Labs

- **GDM**: Two-step glucose test: 50 g glucose followed by 1-hour serum glucose test. Abnormal is >130 to 140 mg/dL, which would then require 3-hour test.
- **Pregestational DM**: Fasting blood glucose > 125 mg/dL, HbA1C ≥ 6.5%, urinalysis > 0.8 mmol/L

Diagnostic Testing

- Biophysical profile (BPP) surveillance to monitor fetal well-being
- Growth ultrasounds to monitor fetal growth
- NSTs to monitor fetal well-being

Treatment

- **GDM treatment**: Diet or medication
- **Pregestational DM**: Medication (insulin required for type 1 pregestational DM)
- **Intrapartum management of GDM and pregestational DM**: May require insulin

Nursing Interventions

- Administer and monitor insulin therapy as indicated and ordered by provider.
- Monitor blood glucose per facility policy.
- Monitor carbohydrate intake.
- Monitor for signs and symptoms of hypoglycemia and hyperglycemia.
- Monitor fetal status per facility policy.

Patient Education

- Monitor blood glucose.
- Recognize signs and symptoms of low and high blood glucose.
- Maintain balanced, low-carbohydrate, limited-sugar diet, and regular exercise.
- See a registered dietician if needed.

ALERT

Teach newly diagnosed patients with GDM the steps for correcting hypoglycemia:
- Sit or lie down in a safe place.
- Eat or drink something sugary, such as 4 oz of regular fruit juice, a half a can of regular soda, 1 tablespoon of sugar, or four glucose tablets.

ALERT

A patient with pregestational diabetes will need close glucose monitoring after delivery because of possible fluctuations in glucose levels. A patient with gestational diabetes will need glucose monitored once after delivery and again in 4 to 12 weeks and should be referred to a primary care provider.

NURSING PEARLS

Educate the patient about the importance of breastfeeding. Breastfeeding can lower the patient's chance of developing type 2 DM by helping the body process glucose and insulin better. Breastfeeding for 2 months has been shown to lower the risk by 50%, and that risk decreases even more after breastfeeding for 5 months.

ALERT

A newborn of a patient with diabetes will need glucose monitoring per institution protocol. The newborn is at risk of hypoglycemia.

POP QUIZ 2.1

A patient is admitted to the labor and delivery triage unit. The patient is approximately 32 weeks pregnant and has had no prenatal care. The patient is complaining of fatigue, excessive urination, and general malaise. The patient thinks it might be a UTI. The initial lab work shows a fasting glucose of 175. What plan of care should the nurse anticipate?

TYPE 1 DIABETES

Overview
- DM type 1 is caused by an environmental or immunologic response in an individual who has a genetic predisposition and has experienced an autoimmune destruction of cells that resulted in hyperglycemia and then complete dependence upon insulin.

Signs and Symptoms
- Dysuria
- Excessive thirst
- Blurred vision
- Fatigue
- Recurrent infections
- Increased hunger
- Unexplained weight loss

Diagnosis
Labs
- Fasting plasma glucose
- Hemoglobin A1C (HgA1c)
- Low-density lipoprotein (LDL)
- Cholesterol

Diagnostic Testing
- 2-hour oral glucose tolerance test
- BP monitoring
- Nonstress test (NST)/BPP BID
- Doppler blood flow studies
- Contraction stress test

Treatment
- Antenatal fetal surveillance up to two times per week
- Monitoring of BP
- Monitoring of blood glucose and HgA1C trends

Nursing Interventions
- Monitor fetal heart rate (FHR) tracing.
- Monitor blood glucose levels.
- Monitor BP.
- Administer metformin or insulin as ordered.

Patient Education
- If you are a smoker, stop smoking.
- Monitor BP at home, noting trends.
- Eat a well-balanced diet and get regular exercise.
- Monitor glucose at home.
- Take medications as prescribed.
- Follow up for weekly NST/BPP. ▶

Patient Education (*continued*)
- Report signs of infections immediately to provider.
- Report signs of depression or anxiety associated with having a long-term disease.

TYPE 2 DIABETES

Overview
- DM type 2 is the most common type of diabetes. It begins with insulin resistance, in which the cells in the pancreas lack the normal efficiency in using insulin, and then it progressively results in an insulin secretory defect.

Signs and Symptoms
- Dysuria
- Excessive thirst
- Blurred vision
- Fatigue
- Recurrent infections
- Sores that do not heal quickly
- Numbness or tingling in hands and/or feet

Diagnosis
Labs
- Fasting plasma glucose
- HgA1C
- LDL
- Cholesterol

Diagnostic Testing
- 2-hour oral glucose tolerance test
- BP monitoring
- NST/BPP BID
- Doppler blood flow studies
- Contraction stress test

Treatment
- Antenatal fetal surveillance up to two times per week
- Monitoring of BP
- Monitoring of blood glucose and HgA1C trends

Nursing Interventions
- Monitor FHR tracing.
- Monitor blood glucose levels.
- Monitor BP.
- Administer metformin or insulin as ordered.
- Manage cholesterol intake.

Patient Education
- If you are a smoker, stop smoking.
- Monitor BP at home, noting trends.
- Get regular exercise. ▶

Patient Education (*continued*)
- Monitor glucose at home.
- Take medications as prescribed.
- Follow up for weekly NST/BPP.
- Report signs of infections immediately to provider.
- Report signs of diabetes distress associated with having long-term disease.

HYPOTHYROIDISM
Overview
- Hypothyroidism is characterized as inadequate thyroid secretion. Patients who have disseminated intravascular coagulation (DIC) are at risk of Hashimoto disease.

Signs and Symptoms
- Fatigue
- Intolerance to cold
- Weight gain
- Nonreassuring fetal heart tracing
- Hair loss, dry skin, and edema
- Muscle spasms or cramping
- Constipation

Diagnosis
Labs
- TSH
- Thyroxine (T4)

Treatment
- Levothyroxine

Nursing Interventions
- Screen infant for hypothyroidism: large tongue, hypotonia, depressed reflexes.
- Monitor fetal well-being.
- Monitor for signs and symptoms of preeclampsia.
- Monitor for postpartum hemorrhage after delivery.

Patient Education
- Monitoring for fetal well-being.
- Take medication as prescribed.
- Go the lab for frequent TSH lab draws.
- Report any new or changing symptoms.
- With history of Graves' disease with treatment, test for TSH receptor antibodies (TRAB) antibodies, as there is a risk of passing it on the fetus.
- Consult with endocrinology as needed throughout pregnancy.

COMPLICATIONS
Patients with hypothyroidism have an increased risk for preeclampsia, placental abruption, Cesarean section, postpartum hemorrhage, low birth weight, preterm or still-born infants.

ALERT!
Levothyroxine should not be taken with prenatal vitamins or other vitamin supplements because the vitamins impair absorption. They should be taken at least 4 hours apart.

HYPERTHYROIDISM

Overview

- Hyperthyroidism occurs when the thyroid produces excess thyroid hormone. Graves disease is the most common cause of hyperthyroidism in patients 20 to 40 years old.
- **Normal changes of pregnancy can mimic hyperthyroidism**: Increase in serum thyroxine-binding globin and increase of thyrotropin (thyroxine-stimulating hormone receptor)
- Treatment is ideal prior to conception.

Signs and Symptoms

- Anxiety, irritability, difficulty sleeping, and nervousness
- Weakness in upper arms and thighs
- Tremors
- Perspiration and intolerance to hot climate
- Fatigue
- Weight loss
- Palpitations and hypertension
- Goiter
- Frequent bowel movements

Diagnosis

Labs
- TSH
- Total triiodothyronine (T3) and T4
- Free T4

Treatment

- Propylthiouracil
- Methimazole

Nursing Interventions

- Monitor vitals (HR over 100).
- Prevent weight loss or failure to gain weight despite adequate nutrition.
- Monitor for heat intolerance.
- Assess eyes for protrusion.
- Monitor fetal heart rating and uterine contraction (UC) pattern.

Patient Education

- Take medication as prescribed.
- Monitor fetal movement.
- Go the lab for frequent TSH lab draws.
- Report any new or changing symptoms.
- Monitor weight loss or gain.
- Know that consultation with endocrinology may be needed throughout pregnancy.

GASTROINTESTINAL SYSTEM

CHOLELITHIASIS

Overview

- Gallstones are more common in pregnant than in nonpregnant patients.
- **Cholelithiasis is classified as either noncomplicated biliary colic or complicated**: cholecystitis (inflammation of the gallbladder), choledocholithiasis, gangrenous gallbladder, pancreatitis.
- Hormonal changes during pregnancy promote gallstone formation. Estrogen increases cholesterol secretion, so more bile is saturated with cholesterol. Progesterone increases, which slows gallbladder emptying, causing bile stasis.
- Acute cholecystitis is a syndrome of right upper quadrant pain, fever, gallbladder inflammation, and leukocytosis.

Signs and Symptoms

- Epigastric pain, particularly in the right upper quadrant
- Pain onset usually 1 to 3 hours postprandial
- Recurrent pain attacks (biliary colic)
- Fever, nausea, vomiting, and anorexia (acute cholecystitis)

Diagnosis

Labs
- CBC
- AST/ALT
- Amylase
- Lipase
- Urine protein

Diagnostic Testing
- Abdominal ultrasound

Treatment

- Nonoperative management
- Operative management for complicated gallstone disease

Nursing Interventions

- Assess pain intensity, location, and aggravating and relieving factors.
- Encourage well-balanced diet and hydration.
- Monitor temperature at regular intervals.
- Initiate antibiotic therapy when appropriate.
- Monitor fetal well-being.

Patient Education

- Avoid eating during painful episodes.
- Monitor fetal movement.
- Take medications as directed.

CHOLESTASIS

Overview

- Intrahepatic cholestasis of pregnancy is the most common type of liver disease in pregnant patients, developing in the second and third trimesters. In this condition, bile accumulates in the blood. Bile acids easily cross the placenta and may begin to accumulate in the fetus. Bile acid accumulation on the fetal side may cause intrauterine demise, meconium-stained amniotic fluid, preterm delivery, and neonatal respiratory distress.

Signs and Symptoms

- **Pruritis**: Common on palms of hand or soles of feet, worsening at night.
- Nausea/anorexia
- Fatigue
- Right upper quadrant abdominal pain
- Dark urine
- Pale stool
- Clinical jaundice (rare but occurs in 1 to 4 weeks after pruritis begins)

Diagnosis

- Based on the presence of pruritis in the third trimester along with elevated total maternal serum bile acids.

Labs

- Serum total bile concentration
- ALT/AST

Treatment

- Upon diagnosis, immediate treatment necessary to decrease maternal symptoms and reduce incidence of perinatal morbidity and mortality
- Ursodeoxycholic acid
- Rifampin
- Cholestyramine
- S-adenosyl-L-methionine

Nursing Interventions

- Administer medication as prescribed.
- Conduct biweekly biophysical profiles and NSTs.
- Prepare patient for induction of labor.
- Monitor fetal well-being.
- Monitor for meconium-stained amniotic fluid in labor.

Patient Education

- Monitor fetal status.
- Take medications as prescribed.
- Follow up with provider for symptoms that worsen.

FATTY LIVER

Overview

- Acute fatty liver of pregnancy (AFLP) is an obstetric emergency, requiring prompt delivery and supportive care for optimal maternal recovery. AFLP is characterized by maternal liver dysfunction or failure and affects other organs as well.
- It is a relatively rare condition that usually occurs in the third trimester.
- Due to symptoms and presentation, it is often confused with preeclampsia, HELLP syndrome, intrahepatic cholestasis, or acute viral hepatitis.

Signs and Symptoms

- **Vague initial symptoms:** nausea, vomiting, abdominal pain, malaise, excessive fatigue
- Jaundice
- Ascites
- Encephalopathy
- Disseminated intravascular coagulopathy
- Hypoglycemia
- Loss of appetite
- Right upper epigastric pain
- Altered level of consciousness
- Polydipsia/polyuria

Diagnosis

Labs
- CBC
- PT/PTT/international normalized ratio (INR)
- Creatinine
- Urine protein (protein: creatinine ratio or 24-hour protein)
- Chemistry (glucose)
- Bilirubin
- AST/ALT

Diagnostic Testing
- Ultrasound
- CT of abdomen

Nursing Interventions

- Prepare patient for delivery.
- Assess postpartum bleeding.
- Maintain strict intake and output.
- Monitor level of consciousness.
- Monitor I/O.
- Monitor blood glucose levels for hypoglycemia.
- Monitor for signs of liver rupture.
- Transfer patient to tertiary care center for delivery and monitoring.
- Monitor fetal heart tracing.

Patient Education
- Know that there will be frequent blood sugar testing and blood draws.
- Know that you will be on continuous fetal monitoring during delivery.
- Report increasing abdominal/right upper quadrant (RUQ) pain.
- Know that you may deliver by emergency Cesarean section.

OBESITY
Overview
- Pregnant patients with obesity may be at risk for gestational hypertension, preeclampsia, gestational diabetes, preterm birth, large-for-gestational-age infants, shoulder dystocia, early pregnancy loss, congenital anomalies, or Cesarean delivery.

Diagnosis
Labs
- **For risks mentioned in Overview**: CBC, glucose, protein creatinine ratio, AST/ALT liver enzymes

Diagnostic Testing
- Fetal surveillance for fetal issues
- Ultrasounds for congenital anomalies

Nursing Interventions
- Use appropriate equipment for patients with obesity (e.g., appropriate-size BP cuff).
- Obtain continuous fetal monitoring, if possible.
- Use maternal pulse oximetry to capture both maternal and FHRs.
- Provide a calm environment and comfort measures.
- Learn patients' pain management plans and communicate with anesthesiologist.
- Assess for cardiopulmonary disease.
- Assess for snoring, hypoxia, and daytime sleepiness.
- Monitor for signs and symptoms of preeclampsia or hyperglycemia.

Patient Education
- Plan to begin breastfeeding shortly after birth.
- Know the signs and symptoms of preeclampsia.

PREGNANCY AFTER BARIATRIC SURGERY
Overview
- Patients who plan to conceive and have received bariatric surgery have increased nutritional needs due to malabsorption of nutrients.
- There is increased risk for intrauterine growth restriction and small-for-gestational-age infants.
- Patients should wait at least 2 years after surgery before conceiving.

Signs and Symptoms
- Nausea, vomiting, and abdominal pain could complicate pregnancy.

Diagnosis

Labs
- Iron
- Folate
- Vitamin B_{12}
- Vitamins A, B, D, and K
- Albumin

Treatment
- Routine prenatal care to closely monitor lab values, nutritional deficiencies, and fetal growth

Nursing Interventions
- Provide nutritional supplementation as appropriate.
- Monitor for changes in gastrointestinal system such as abdominal pain and new-onset GI discomfort.
- Monitor fetal well-being.
- Monitor for signs and symptoms of hyperemesis.
- Monitor blood glucose as appropriate.

Patient Education
- Eat small, frequent meals.
- Report new-onset GI issues to the provider, including dumping syndrome.
- Monitor fetal activity.
- Take medications as prescribed.
- Monitor blood glucose as appropriate.

HEMATOPOETIC ANEMIA

Overview
- There are two common types of anemia in pregnancy, physiologic anemia and iron deficiency anemia. Physiologic anemia occurs when maternal physiologic changes result in diluted blood. Plasma volume and red blood cell mass increases, causing mild anemia. Iron-deficiency anemia occurs when the patient does not get enough iron in the diet, does not absorb iron well, has had a short interval between pregnancies, or has lost blood in pregnancies or menstruation.
- Fetal risks due to maternal anemia are low birth weight and premature birth.

Signs and Symptoms
- Fatigue
- Weakness
- Pallor or yellow-tinted skin
- Vertigo
- Tachycardia

Diagnosis

Labs
- CBC
- Ferritin

Treatment

- Oral iron for those who can tolerate it.
- IV iron for severe anemia, patients who cannot tolerate oral iron, or no hemoglobin (Hg) increase with oral use

Nursing Interventions

- Monitor vital signs regularly.
- Measure blood loss.
- Assess skin and capillary refill.

Patient Education

- Know that it takes 2 weeks for oral iron to effectively increase hemoglobin molecules.
- Consult with dietary/nutrition resources as needed.

DISSEMINATED INTRAVASCULAR COAGULATION (DIC)

Overview

- DIC is a serious disorder that causes abnormal blood clotting that blocks blood vessels. The normal blood clotting process becomes overactive, destroying organs.
- Pregnancy is a hypercoagulable state that prevents excess bleeding during placenta separation. Abnormal activation of this state can result in microvascular thrombosis, endothelial damage, hemorrhage, and organ failure.

Signs and Symptoms

- Uterine bleeding
- Bleeding from gums, catheter, IV sites, and venipuncture sites
- Spontaneous bruising
- Petechiae
- Signs of shock (tachycardia, hypotension, weak peripheral pulses, altered mental status)

Diagnosis

Labs

- CBC (thrombocytopenia)
- Clotting factors (activated partial thromboplastin clotting time [aPTT], PT, INR)
- Fibrinogen
- D-dimer

Treatment

- Identify and address the event that triggered DIC (pre-eclampsia, sepsis, placental abruption, postpartum hemorrhage).
- Identify those patients at risk of DIC.

Nursing Interventions

- Ensure patient has two large-bore IV sites.
- Assess HR, BP, temperature, mental status, and skin.
- Maintain MAP of greater than or equal to 65.
- Apply Bair Hugger.
- Measure strict I/Os. Immediately report of urine output <30 mL per hour.
- Have blood type and screen ready. ▶

Nursing Interventions (*continued*)
- Administer blood products to achieve euvolemia.
- Prepare for mass transfusion.
- Assess continuous FHR.
- Notify provider of FHR trends and immediately notify of category 3 tracing.
- Monitor underlying cause (e.g., preeclampsia, eclampsia, hemorrhage, sepsis)

Patient Education
- Report difficulty breathing or pounding heart.
- Know that you may need transfer to a tertiary care center.
- Know that you may need multiple blood transfusions.
- Know that you may need admission to the ICU and separation from newborn.
- Know that the newborn may need NICU admission

HEMOLYTIC DISEASE
Overview
- Sickle cell disease is a common genetic disorder that causes red blood cells to have a sickled shape with low oxygen-carrying capacity. These abnormally shaped red blood cells clump together in the blood vessels and prevent oxygen from being delivered to other parts of the body.
- Thalassemias are genetic blood disorders that cause anemia. They can be referred to as alpha or beta, depending on the changes made within the hemoglobin.

Signs and Symptoms
- **Sickle cell anemia**: pain generalized and in joints, infection, anemia, jaundice, fatigue, shortness of breath, stroke, and issues with organs such as lungs, spleen, and kidney
- **Thalassemias**: Patients may be asymptomatic with mild forms of thalassemia. More severe forms may have anemia and issues with organs such as the heart, spleen, and bone.

Diagnosis
- Sickle cell disease diagnostic testing is normally performed within the first 24 to 48 hours after birth with the newborn screening test. Screening can also be done in childhood with the hemoglobin S or sickle hemoglobin blood test and genetic testing to determine if the individual is a carrier versus having the disease.
- Thalassemia diagnosis is normally done in childhood, prior to the age of 2 years when symptoms normally present. It can be tested later with lab tests including CBC, reticulocyte count, iron levels, hemoglobin electrophoresis, and genetic testing.

Labs
- **Sickle cell** disease: Blood test for the hemoglobin S or sickle hemoglobin, hemoglobin electrophoresis, carrier test for partners of sickle cell carriers
- **Thalassemia**: CBC, reticulocyte count, iron levels, hemoglobin electrophoresis, genetic testing

Treatment
- **For both sickle cell disease and thalassemia**: Obstetrician and hematology specialist may work together in pregnancy management.
- **Sickle cell disease**: Frequent prenatal visits, IV hydration, pain medication, hydroxyurea (prevents complications of sickle cell disease) are necessary.
- **Thalassemia**: Medications, blood transfusions, frequent prenatal visits are necessary.

Nursing Interventions

- Monitor pain.
- Monitor fetal well-being.
- Administer medications as directed.
- Monitor for signs of preeclampsia, eclampsia, and gestational hypertension.
- Monitor for signs of placental abruption.
- Monitor for pain or symptoms associated with urinary tract infection (UTI)/ kidney stones/gallstones.

Patient Education

- Know that you may need blood transfusions during pregnancy to treat anemia.
- Monitor fetal movement during pregnancy.
- Report any new signs or symptoms or changes immediately.
- Take medications as directed.
- Monitor for and report signs of preeclampsia.
- Report pain in abdomen or back from kidney or gallstones.
- Report any signs of UTI.
- Come to hospital for vaginal bleeding or abdominal pain.
- Take over-the-counter acetaminophen or ibuprofen for mild pain.
- Drink plenty of fluids.
- Avoid situations or stressors that would trigger a crisis.

THROMBOCYTOPENIA

Overview

- Identifying the cause of thrombocytopenia can help guide management. Possible causes of thrombocytopenia are gestational thrombocytopenia, immune thrombocytopenia, drug induced, preeclampsia, HELLP syndrome, disseminated intravascular coagulation, acute fatty liver, thrombotic microangiopathy, TTP, complement-mediated thrombotic microangiopathy (TMA), or Shiga toxin–mediated hemolytic uremic syndrome.
- Thrombocytopenia is defined as low platelet count, typically <100,000/mcL.

Signs and Symptoms

- Easy or excessive bruising
- Bleeding from gums or nose
- Petechiae
- Blood in urine or stools

Diagnosis

Labs
- CBC
- Peripheral blood smear

Treatment

- Platelet transfusion
- **Immune Thrombocytopenia (ITP)**: steroids (take a few days to have an effect), IVIG, splenectomy (if not responsive to the first line of treatment)

Nursing Interventions
- Monitor for signs of infection.
- Avoid fetal scalp electrode (FSE) for maternal platelet count <80,000.
- Collect blood samples for laboratory evaluation to reach platelet goal of >80,000.
- Monitor fetal well-being.
- Monitor bleeding.

Patient Education
- Avoid nonsteroidal anti-inflammatory medications.
- Avoid salicylates unless low dose for pre-eclampsia.
- Avoid trauma.
- Report bleeding that is not stopping.
- Get frequent lab draws for platelets.
- Monitor fetal movement.

THROMBOPHILIA

Overview
- Inherited thrombophilias are genetic conditions that increase the risk of thromboembolic events. Pregnancy is a hypercoagulable state, and thrombophilia increases maternal opportunities for venous thrombosis and pulmonary embolism. Patients who are pregnant and who have thrombophilia are at increased risk of pregnancy loss, fetal growth restriction, late miscarriage, placental abruption, preeclampsia, and stillbirths.

Signs and Symptoms
- **Deep vein thrombosis (DVT) in extremity:** inflammation, pain, swelling, warmth, redness
- **Pulmonary embolism (depends on size/location):** feeling of doom, dyspnea, tachypnea, productive cough, rales on pulmonary auscultation

Diagnosis
Labs
- Antiphospholipid antibodies if no history

Diagnostic Testing
- Chest x-ray
- CT or ventilation/perfusion scan with contrast
- Angiography
- MRI
- Doppler ultrasound of vein

Treatment
- Anticoagulants such as heparin with a larger dose postpartum

Nursing Interventions
- Provide early respiratory support and cardiac support if needed.
- Monitor for shortness of breath and chest pain.
- Monitor for signs and symptoms of DVT.
- Place pneumatic compression devices prior to Cesarean section. ▶

Nursing Interventions (*continued*)
- Encourage early ambulation after Cesarean section.
- Administer medications as directed.

Patient Education
- Know that delivery will be scheduled at 39 weeks' gestation.
- Know that pneumatic compression devices are placed before Cesarean section and worn afterward.
- Know that you will walk soon after Cesarean section to prevent blood clots.
- Know that anticoagulants will be restarted 4 to 12 hours after delivery.
- Report SOB, chest pain, or redness and pain in lower extremity.

INFECTIOUS DISEASE BACTERIAL VAGINOSIS (BV)

Overview
- Bacterial vaginosis is an overgrowth of normal vaginal bacteria and is common in 20% of pregnancies.

Signs and Symptoms
- Fishy-smelling vaginal discharge
- Thin white or gray discharge
- Vaginal itching or burning or pain
- Burning with urination

Diagnosis
Diagnostic Testing
- Wet mount prep of vaginal secretions

Treatment
- Metronidazole
- Clindamycin

Nursing Interventions
- Monitor for premature rupture of membranes (PROM)/preterm labor.
- Monitor for increased temperature during labor (chorioamnionitis).
- Monitor for postpartum endometritis and pain.

Patient Education
- Do not use douching products.
- Know that untreated BV may lead to preterm birth or low-birth-weight infant.
- Take all medication as prescribed, even if asymptomatic.
- Be tested for HIV and other STIs.
- Return to provider if symptoms persist despite treatment.
- Go to the labor and delivery (L&D) department for PROM or preterm labor.
- Monitor fetal movement.
- Report to provider any foul-smelling discharge and abdominal pain after delivery.
- Know that metronidazole is excreted in breast milk so you may need to defer breastfeeding for 12 to 24 hours after treatment, depending on dose.

COVID-19

Overview

- COVID-19–positive pregnant patients may be asymptomatic or symptomatic. Asymptomatic patients typically have a better sequalae than symptomatic patients.
- Vaccination reduces the severity of the disease and is safe in pregnant patients.

Signs and Symptoms

- Fatigue
- Shortness of breath
- Congestion
- Headache
- Nausea and vomiting

Diagnosis

Labs

- Nasopharyngeal swab for viral antigens

Diagnostic Testing

- Chest x-ray

Treatment

- **Asymptomatic patients**: hydration, rest, ambulation, supportive measures
- **Symptomatic patients**: steroids, antiviral drugs, anticoagulant, monoclonal antibodies, dexamethasone, nirmatrelvir-ritonavir, or remdesivir

Nursing Interventions

- Place sequential compression device (SCD) on patient when not ambulating.
- Monitor vital signs including temperature and respiratory rate.
- Titrate oxygen administration to achieve SpO_2 greater than 94%.
- Place patient in prone positioning for severe respiratory symptoms.
- Monitor blood sugar in patients receiving steroids.

Patient Education

- Wear a mask indoors in public places.
- Report to provider if oxygen saturation is less than 94%.
- Report SOB/chest pain.
- Monitor fetal well-being.
- Wash hands with soap and water often.
- Stay 6 feet from others.
- Call 911 if you need emergent help.

CHLAMYDIA

Overview

- *Chlamydia trachomatis* is the most common sexually transmitted genital infection. The majority of infected people are asymptomatic, causing an ongoing infection source. Newborns delivered vaginally by an infected patient can develop chlamydia, conjunctivitis, and pneumonia. Chlamydia infections often accompany gonorrhea. Screening is indicated for all pregnant patients.

Signs and Symptoms

- Often asymptomatic
- Change in vaginal discharge
- Intermenstrual vaginal bleeding
- Postcoital bleeding

Diagnosis

Labs

- Nucleic acid amplification testing: swab or urine

Treatment

- Amoxicillin
- Azithromycin
- Expedited partner therapy

Nursing Interventions

- Monitor for signs of preterm labor.
- If newborn is positive for chlamydia, monitor for pneumonia and conjunctivitis.

Patient Education

- Do not have sexual intercourse for 7 days once treatment is started.
- Have follow-up testing 3 months after treatment.
- Use condoms with new partners or when in nonmonogamous relationships.
- Advise sexual partners to be tested as well.
- Return if symptomatic despite treatment.

GONORRHEA

Overview

- Gonorrhea is the second most reported communicable disease. Patients may take up to 10 days to start developing symptoms.

Signs and Symptoms

- Vaginal itching
- Burning with urination
- Yellowish vaginal discharge
- Bleeding

Diagnosis

Diagnostic Testing

- **Nucleic acid amplification testing:** swab or urine

Treatment

- Ceftriaxone

Nursing Interventions

- Monitor fetal well-being and fetal movement.

Patient Education

- Have follow-up testing 3 months after treatment.
- Notify other sexual partners to be treated.
- Take all medications as prescribed.
- Follow up with provider if symptomatic despite treatment.
- Know that you may need to be rescreened in the third trimester if high risk.

GROUP BETA STREP (GBS)

Overview

- Group B *Streptococcus* (GBS) is found in the genital or gastrointestinal tracts of adults. Pregnant patients with GBS are often asymptomatic.

COMPLICATIONS

Fetus is at risk for vertical transmission if the mother is untreated. The neonate can be at risk for congenital pneumonia, early onset GBS infection, and/or sepsis/meningitis

Signs and Symptoms

- Possible UTI or back pain

Diagnosis

- Group Beta strep is diagnosed by using a cotton swab to collect a sample from the vagina and the rectum to determine if it cultures positive for Group Beta strep.

Labs

- Urine culture or vaginal-rectal culture

Treatment

- Penicillin G or other antibiotic in case of allergy

Nursing Interventions

- Administer antibiotics as scheduled for patients with unknown GBS status or positive status.
- Collect specimen prior to digital exam or speculum exam.

Patient Education

- Notify nurse and provider of positive GBS upon admission.

HERPES

Overview

- Genital herpes simplex virus (HSV) is common. Infection occurs when there is skin or mucous membrane contact with an active lesion.
- The virus migrates to sensory nerves and becomes latent. It can be reactivated and become a recurrent infection.
- Vertical transmission can occur when membranes are ruptured and the virus ascends from an active lesion or during birth when the fetus comes in contact with an active lesion.

Signs and Symptoms

- Fever
- Malaise
- Myalgia
- Dysuria ▶

Signs and Symptoms (*continued*)
- Local pain and itching
- Tender lymphadenopathy

Diagnosis
Labs
- Viral culture
- PCR

Treatment
- Acyclovir or valacyclovir orally at 36 weeks to suppress the virus
- C-section delivery in the presence of active lesions recommended

Nursing Interventions
- Labor is a stressor; monitor for development of lesions during labor.
- Assess last acyclovir administration.

Patient Education
- Take medication as prescribed.
- Notify provider if membranes rupture prior to labor.
- Notify provider if you notice a lesion developing.
- Ensure sexual partners are treated.

HIV INFECTION

Overview
- HIV is an infection that reduces the body's ability to fight off infection and is the virus that leads to AIDS. HIV is spread through contact with bodily fluids, such as blood or semen. It may also be transmitted vertically from the pregnant patient to the fetus or perinatally during birth or with breastfeeding. With routine screening prenatally and positive cases treated with antiretroviral therapy (ART), the risk of spreading HIV to the fetus or newborn is greatly reduced.

Signs and Symptoms
- There may be no signs of infection early on, and many patients will not know they have HIV until they become sick.
- When infection is present and active, fever and thrush are common early signs.

Diagnosis
Labs
- HIV is diagnosed by a HIV-1 antigen or HIV-2 antibody blood test.
- Routine screening is done using a blood sample, generally at the first prenatal visit.
- The screening test detects the presence of the HIV-1 antigen or HIV-2 antibodies.

Diagnostic Testing
- HIV infection is monitored during pregnancy by measuring the CD4 count, or percentage of CD4, and by monitoring the viral load.

Treatment
- Treatment should begin early in pregnancy to minimize the risk of transmission to the fetus.
- ART is a combination of various drugs to combat the retrovirus. Because these drugs can become toxic, regular testing is done to assess the pregnant patient's tolerance and to adjust the drugs if necessary.

Nursing Interventions
- Monitor fetal well-being.
- If patient is in labor, administer rapid point of care testing for HIV if not previously done.
- Administer antiretroviral prophylaxis in labor or prior to Cesarean section.
- Use standard precautions, and monitor for signs of infection.
- Assess for postpartum depression.

Patient Education
- Know that regular testing will be done throughout pregnancy to assess the level of infection and adjust treatment as appropriate.
- Know that your provider will discuss the best method of delivery and if early delivery is recommended based on viral load and CD4 counts.
- Avoid breastfeeding because the virus can be spread through breast milk.
- Know that carefully following the prescribed ART, delivering by Cesearean section, and not breastfeeding minimize the chance of passing the virus to the infant.

HUMAN PAPILLOMAVIRUS (HPV)

Overview
- HPV is a viral infection and is the most common STI. It causes an overgrowth of intraepithelial cells and is also known as genital warts. It has been found to increase the risk of cervical cancer if untreated.

Signs and Symptoms
- Often none
- Appearance of genital or rectal warts
- Cervical bleeding

Diagnosis
Diagnostic Testing
- HPV is diagnosed by sampling scrapings of cervical cellst
- It is diagnostic if warts are visualized.

Treatment
- Removal of warts can be done by freezing or excision as an office procedure.
- Routine monitoring of abnormal cervical cells should be done if noted on screening. There is no treatment for HPV, but routine monitoring provides for early recognition and treatment of cervical cancer.

Patient Education
- Know that follow-up testing is important.
- Notify sexual partners to get follow-up and examination.

INFLUENZA
Overview

- Pregnant patients and those who are in the postpartum period are at increased risk of severe complications related to seasonal influenza as well as pandemic influenza infections. Influenza infections can create a multitude of health issues for the already at-risk pregnant patient. Patients who have underlying health problems are at greater risk of influenza-related risks. Patients should be treated within 48 hours of symptoms and up to 2 weeks in postpartum period.

Signs and Symptoms

- Fever >100.0°F: may or may not be present
- Cough
- Fatigue
- Headache
- Generalized body aches

Diagnosis

Diagnostic Testing

- Rapid influenza diagnostic test (false-negative tests common)
- Molecular influenza diagnostic test
- Rapid antigen testing-polymerase chain reaction and viral culture

Treatment

Patients suspected of having influenza or with confirmed influenza: Treat with antivirals:

- Oseltamivir (first-line treatment)
- Zanamivir
- Acetaminophen for fever

Nursing Interventions

- Administer medications as prescribed.
- Monitor for fever.
- Monitor fetal well-being.
- Report any changes in condition to provider.
- Administer IV hydration as needed.

Patient Education

- Go to the emergency department or labor and delivery if unable to hold down fluids, if experiencing shortness of breath or chest pain, or if having pregnancy-related issues such as decreased fetal movement.
- Take all medications as prescribed; know that family members will also need to be treated for influenza.

ZIKA VIRUS
Overview

- The Zika virus can be transmitted from a mosquito bite or from sexual intercourse with someone infected with virus, even if they are asymptomatic.

Signs and Symptoms

- Fever
- Generalized rash ▶

Signs and Symptoms (*continued*)
- Generalized joint or muscle pain
- Reddened eyes
- Headache

Diagnosis
Diagnostic Testing
- Molecular testing of blood and urine for presences of the virus

Treatment/Prevention
- Thorough wash hands.
- Avoid traveling to areas with known Zika virus infections.

Nursing Interventions
- Clean and disinfect all surfaces that were exposed to Zika.
- Monitor fetal well-being.

Patient Education
- Monitor fetal well-being/kick counts.
- Clean and disinfect all surfaces.
- Notify provider for immediate testing if you have traveled where Zika exposure is likely.
- Notify your provider if you have signs and symptoms after travel.

SYPHILIS
Overview
- Syphilis is caused by bacteria that enters the body through a cut in the skin or through contact with a partner's syphilis sore called a chancre. Syphilis is most commonly spread through sexual contact.

Signs and Symptoms
- Chancre
- Rash on soles of feet and palms of hands
- Flat warts on vulva
- Flu-like symptoms

Diagnosis
- Diagnosis is based upon sexual history, signs and symptoms, and diagnostic testing.

Diagnostic Testing
- Rapid plasma reagin (RPR)_
- Venereal disease research laboratory (VDRL)
- Automated Tripoemal test (enzyme immunoassay [EIA], chemiluminescence immunoassay [CIA])

Treatment
- Pregnant patients who are diagnosed with syphilis should be treated with a penicillin regimen immediately upon diagnosis.

Nursing Interventions

- Monitor for preterm labor/fetal distress.
- Administer medication as prescribed.

Patient Education

- Take all medications as prescribed.
- Follow up with provider as scheduled.
- Advise sexual partner(s) to be treated.
- Monitor fetal well-being.

URINARY TRACT INFECTION (UTI)

Overview

- A UTI is a common infection in which bacteria enter into the urinary tract, which includes the bladder (cystitis), urethra (urethritis), ureters, and kidney (pyelonephritis).

Signs and Symptoms

- Urgency
- Urinary frequency
- Burning or pain with urination
- Blood in urine
- Abdominal or back pain

Diagnosis

Diagnostic Testing
- Urinalysis
- Urine culture

Treatment

- Antibiotics
- Antispasmodics

Nursing Interventions

- Monitor for fetal well-being and preterm labor.
- Monitor for progression of symptoms to pyelonephritis.
- Encourage oral fluids.
- Administer antibiotics as prescribed.
- Monitor urine output.

Patient Education

- Drink plenty of fluids.
- Empty bladder every 2 to 3 hours.
- Take medications as prescribed.
- Report to provider if symptoms are not improved or are worse.
- Monitor fetal well-being and for signs of preterm labor.

MULTIPLE GESTATION

Overview
- A pregnancy that has more than one fetus is considered multiple gestation. Multiple gestation can be the product of one ovum and one sperm that divide into multiple cells or more than one ovum and sperm. This can be caused spontaneously or with the use of fertility medication. Multiple gestation can be monochorionic or dichorionic or a combination of both. The incidence of multiple gestation increases with maternal age.

Management
- The management of multiple gestation depends on chronicity.

Maternal Complications
- Anemia
- Gestational diabetes
- Preeclampsia/eclampsia
- HELLP (may need to transfer to a tertiary care center)
- Preterm labor and delivery
- Postpartum hemorrhage

Fetal Complications
- Stillbirth
- Prematurity
- Cerebral palsy
- Intraventricular hemorrhage
- Neonatal death
- Respiratory distress

Signs and Symptoms
- Severe nausea and vomiting (hyperemesis gravidarum)
- Breast tenderness
- Rapid weight gain

Diagnosis
Diagnostic Testing
- Ultrasound

Treatment
- **Low-dose aspirin:** prophylaxis
- Short-term tocolytics
- Calcium channel blockers
- Nonsteroidal inflammatories
- Corticosteroids
- Antiemetics
- Magnesium sulfate for preeclampsia/neuroprotection
- Cerclage if needed
- Cervical length/fetal fibronectin
- Scheduled delivery starting at 32 weeks, depending on chronicity

Nursing Interventions

- Monitor fetal well-being.
- Administer medications as prescribed.
- Monitor for signs and symptoms of preterm labor/preeclampsia/HELLP/eclampsia.
- Monitor I/O closely if patient is taking magnesium sulfate or has hyperemesis.
- Monitor blood sugars.

Patient Education

- Consume 300 extra calories per day per fetus.
- Stay active but avoid strenuous exercise.
- Know that you will have more frequent appointments with your provider.
- Report signs and symptoms of preeclampsia or preterm labor.
- Monitor fetal status.
- Know that you may need a Cesarean delivery.

AMNIOTIC FLUID ASSESSMENT OLIGOHYDRAMNIOS

Overview

- In oligohydramnios, there is less than normal amniotic fluid surrounding the fetus, a single pocket contains approximately 2 cm or less, and there is a total amniotic fluid index (AFI) of equal to or less than 5 cm in all total pockets. The normal amount of amniotic fluid is greater than 5 cm to less than 24 cm of fluid.

Signs and Symptoms

- Leaking or gush of fluid from vagina
- Fetal growth restriction
- Uterine size measuring smaller than normal for gestation
- Decreased fetal movement
- Not gaining enough weight

Diagnosis

Diagnostic Testing

- Ultrasound evaluation of amniotic fluid index or maximum vertical pocket to determine 5 cm or less of amniotic fluid
- Spontaneous rupture of membranes (SROM) to check for ferning, nitrazine, and pooling
- Alpha-fetoprotein

Treatment

- Antenatal surveillance one to two times per week and NST
- Induction of labor
- Amnioinfusion if cord compression in labor

Nursing Interventions

- If using continuous monitoring, monitor for late decelerations or variable decelerations.
- Perform amnioinfusion if there are variable decelerations in labor.
- Perform NST.
- Monitor underlying health issues.

Patient Education
- Drink adequate water.
- Monitor fetal movement.
- Come to L&D if leaking fluid or if there is decreased fetal movement
- Attend appointments for antenatal surveillance and NSTs.
- Report any changes in BP or blood sugars.
- Know that you may need a Cesarean section.

POLYHYDRAMNIOS

Overview
- Polyhydramnios occurs when more than the normal amount of amniotic fluid surrounds the fetus. The normal amount of amniotic fluid is >5 cm to <24 cm of fluid.
- There are different degrees of polyhydramnios: mild (24 to 29.9 cm), moderate (30 to 34.9 cm), and severe (35 cm or greater).

Signs and Symptoms
- Preterm contractions/preterm labor
- Painful contractions
- Tense abdomen
- Preterm premature rupture of membranes (PPROM)
- Placental abruption
- Uterine atony/hemorrhage
- Maternal shortness of breath
- Edema of the lower extremities

Diagnosis
- Ultrasound for AFI and fetal malformations
- Uterine size larger than expected for gestational age

Diagnostic Testing
- Ultrasound every 4 weeks for fetal anatomy scan and fetal size

Treatment
- Delivery at 39 weeks
- Amnioreduction if maternal symptoms are severe

Nursing Interventions
- Monitor fetal well-being.
- Monitor pain.
- Assess for prolapsed cord with rupture of membranes.
- Assess for SOB.
- Assist with amnioreduction.
- Monitor for bleeding associated with placental abruption.

Patient Education
- Notify provider for shortness of breath or lower-extremity edema.
- Go to L&D for spontaneous rupture of membranes (SROM). ▶

Patient Education (*continued*)
- Call 911 if you notice SROM or prolapsed cord.
- Keep scheduled appointments for antenatal surveillance and NST.

APPENDIX 2.1 MEDICATIONS FOR DM IN PREGNANCY

INDICATIONS	MECHANISM OF ACTION	CONTRAINDICATIONS, PRECAUTIONS, AND ADVERSE EFFECTS
Biguanides (metformin)		
• Type 2 DM (First-line treatment)	• Decrease the amount of glucose absorbed from food and the amount of glucose made by the liver • Increase the body's response to insulin	• Contraindications include severe kidney impairment, acute or chronic metabolic acidosis, and hypersensitivity to metformin. • Biguanides can cause lactic acidosis; report new signs of fatigue or muscle aches. • Adverse effects include diarrhea, nausea, vomiting, flatulence, and asthenia.
Sulfonylurea (glyburide)		
• Type 2 DM (Second-line treatment)	• Stimulates insulin release from the pancreatic beta cells • Reduces glucose output from the liver • Increases insulin sensitivity at peripheral target sites	• Contraindications include hypersensitivity to glyburide, type 1 DM, and diabetic ketoacidosis. • Monitor for hypoglycemia. • Adverse effects include epigastric fullness, heartburn, and nausea.
Insulin (aspart, lispro)		
• Type 1 DM • Type 2 DM • Gestational DM	• Rapid acting, shorter lasting • Converts glucose in the blood to energy in cells	• There are no contraindications. • Less risk of hypoglycemia, compared to long-acting insulin. • Dosage should be modified depending on clinical response and degree of hepatic and/or renal impairment.
Insulin (regular)		
• Type 1 DM • Type 2 DM • Gestational DM	• Short acting • Converts glucose in the blood to energy in cells	• There are no contraindications. • Monitor for low blood sugar, follow diet, take appropriate dose, wear medical ID alert, and carry a quick-acting sugar for hypoglycemia. • Adverse effects include hypoglycemia, seizures, weight gain. • Dosage should be modified depending on clinical response and degree of hepatic and/or renal impairment.

(*continued*)

APPENDIX 2.1 MEDICATIONS FOR DM IN PREGNANCY (*continued*)

INDICATIONS	MECHANISM OF ACTION	CONTRAINDICATIONS, PRECAUTIONS, AND ADVERSE EFFECTS
Insulin (NPH)		
• Type 1 DM • Type 2 DM • Gestational DM	• Immediate acting • Converts glucose in the blood to energy in cells.	• There are no contraindications. • Monitor for low blood sugar, follow diet, take appropriate dose, wear medical ID alert, and carry a quick acting sugar for hypoglycemia. • Adverse effects include hypoglycemia, seizures, weight gain. • Dosage should be modified depending on clinical response and degree of hepatic and/or renal impairment.

RESOURCES

ACOG. (2017a). ACOG Practice Bulletin 181: Prevention of Rh D alloimmunization. *Obstetrics & Gynecology, 130*(2), e57–e70. https://doi.org/10.1097/AOG.0000000000002232

ACOG. (2017b). ACOG Practice Bulletin 183: Postpartum hemorrhage. *Obstetrics & Gynecology*, https://www.acog.org/clinical/clinical-guidance/practice-bulletin/articles/2017/10/postpartum-hemorrhage

ACOG. (2018a). Committee Opinion 752: Prenatal and perinatal human immunodeficiency virus testing. *Obstetrics & Gynecology*, https://www.acog.org/clinical/clinical-guidance/committee-opinion/articles/2018/09/prenatal-and-perinatal-human-immunodeficiency-virus-testing

ACOG. (2018b). ACOG Practice Bulletin 132: Anitphospholipid syndrome. *Obstetrics & Gynecology, 120*(6), 1514–1521. https://doi.org/10.1097/01.AOG.0000423816.39542.0f

ACOG. (2018c). ACOG Practice Bulletin 190: Gestational diabetes mellitus. *Obstetrics & Gynecology, 131*(2), 49–64. https://doi.org/10.1097/aog.0000000000002501

ACOG. (2018d). ACOG Practice Bulletin 196: Thromboembolism in pregnancy. *Obstetrics & Gynecology*, https://www.acog.org/clinical/clinical-guidance/practice-bulletin/articles/2018/07/thromboembolism-in-pregnancy

ACOG. (2018e). ACOG Practice Bulletin 197: Inherited thrombophilias in pregnancy. *Obstetrics & Gynecology*, https://www.acog.org/clinical/clinical-guidance/practice-bulletin/articles/2018/07/inherited-thrombophilias-in-pregnancy

ACOG. (2018f). ACOG Practice Bulletin 201: Summary: Pregestational diabetes mellitus. *Obstetrics & Gynecology, 132*(6), 1514–1516. https://doi.org/10.1097/aog.0000000000002961

ACOG. (2019a). ACOG Committee Opinion 831: Medically indicated late preterm and early term deliveries. *Obstetrics & Gynecology*, chrome-extension://efaidnbmnnnibpcajpcglclefindmkaj/https://www.acog.org/-/media/project/acog/acogorg/clinical/files/committee-opinion/articles/2021/07/medically-indicated-late-preterm-and-early-term-deliveries.pdf

ACOG. (2019b). ACOG Practice Bulletin. 202: Gestational hypertension and preeclampsia. *Obstetrics & Gynecology, 133*(1), e1–e25.

ACOG. (2019c). ACOG Practice Bulletin 203: Chronic hypertension in pregnancy. *Obstetrics & Gynecology, 133*(1), e26–e50. https://doi.org/10.1097/AOG.0000000000003020

ACOG. (2019d). ACOG Practice Bulletin 207: Thrombocytopenia in pregnancy. *Obstetrics & Gynecology*, https://www.acog.org/clinical/clinical-guidance/practice-bulletin/articles/2019/03/thrombocytopenia-in-pregnancy

ACOG. (2019e). ACOG Practice Bulletin 212: Pregnancy and heart disease. *Obstetrics & Gynecology, 133*(5), e320–e356. https://doi.org/10.1097/AOG.0000000000003243

ACOG. (2019f). A healthy pregnancy for women with diabetes. *American College of Obstetricians and Gynecologists*. https://www.acog.org/womens-health/faqs/a-healthy-pregnancy-for-women-with-diabetes

ACOG. (2020a). ACOG Committee Opinion 809: Human papillomavirus vaccination. https://www.acog.org/clinical/clinical-guidance/committee-opinion/articles/2020/08/human-papillomavirus-vaccination

ACOG. (2020b). ACOG Practice Bulletin 216: Macrosomia. *Obstetrics & Gynecology*, https://www.acog.org/-/media/project/acog/acogorg/clinical/files/practice-bulletin/articles/2020/01/macrosomia.pdf

ACOG. (2020c). ACOG Practice Bulletin 223: Thyroid disease in pregnancy. *Obstetrics & Gynecology*. https://www.acog.org/-/media/project/acog/acogorg/clinical/files/practice-bulletin/articles/2020/06/thyroid-disease-in-pregnancy.pdf

ACOG. (2021a). ACOG Committee Opinion 828: Indications for outpatient antenatal fetal surveillance. *Obstetrics & Gynecology*, https://www.acog.org/clinical/clinical-guidance/committee-opinion/articles/2021/06/indications-for-outpatient-antenatal-fetal-surveillanceACOG.

ACOG. (2021b). Committee Opinion 753: Assessment and treatment of pregnant women with suspected or confirmed influenza. *Obstetrics & Gynecology*, https://www.acog.org/clinical/clinical-guidance/committee-opinion/articles/2018/10/assessment-and-treatment-of-pregnant-women-with-suspected-or-confirmed-influenza

ACOG. (2021c). ACOG Committee Opinion 828: Indications for outpatient antenatal fetal surveillance. *Obstetrics & Gynecology*, https://www.acog.org/-/media/project/acog/acogorg/clinical/files/committee-opinion/articles/2021/06/indications-for-outpatient-antenatal-fetal-surveillance.pdf

ACOG. (2021d). Gestational diabetes. *Obstetrics & Gynecology*, https://www.acog.org/womens-health/faqs/gestational-diabetes

ACOG. (2021). Group B strep in pregnancy. *Obstetrics & Gynecology*. https://www.acog.org/womens-health/faqs/group-b-strep-and-pregnancy

ACOG. (2021f). Obesity and pregnancy. *Obstetrics & Gynecology*, https://www.acog.org/womens-health/faqs/obesity-and-pregnancy

ACOG. (2021g). Practice Bulletin 231. Multifetal gestations twin, triplet, and higher-order multifetal pregnancies. *Obstetrics & Gynecology*, https://www.acog.org/clinical/clinical-guidance/practice-bulletin/articles/2021/06/multifetal-gestations-twin-triplet-and-higher-order-multifetal-pregnancies

ACOG. (2022a). Carrier screening for hemoglobinopathies: Sickle cell disease and thalassemia. *Obstetrics & Gynecology*, https://www.acog.org/womens-health/faqs/carrier-screening-for-hemoglobinopathies

ACOG. (2022b). Chlamydia, gonorrhea, and syphilis. *Obstetrics & Gynecology*, https://www.acog.org/womens-health/faqs/chlamydia-gonorrhea-and-syphilis

ACOG. (2022c). Multiple gestation. *Obstetrics & Gynecology*, https://www.acog.org/womens-health/faqs/multiple-pregnancy

ACOG. (2022d). Safe motherhood initiative: Severe hypertension. *Obstetrics & Gynecology*, https://www.acog.org/community/districts-and-sections/district-ii/programs-and-resources/safe-motherhood-initiative/severe-hypertension

ACOG. (2022e). Urinary tract infections. *Obstetrics & Gynecology*, https://www.acog.org/womens-health/faqs/urinary-tract-infections

ADA. (2021). *Diabetes and breastfeeding*. https://www.diabetes.org/resources/women/prenatal-care/diabetes-breastfeeding.

American Thyroid Association. (2019). *Hypothyroidism in pregnancy*. https://www.thyroid.org/wp-content/uploads/patients/brochures/hypothyroidism_pregnancy_brochure.pdf

Arthritis.org. (2022). *Rheumatoid arthritis and pregnancy*. https://www.arthritis.org/health-wellness/healthy-living/family-relationships/family-planning/rheumatoid-arthritis-and-pregnancy#:~:text=Womenwho have uncontrolled rheumatoid,medical care early in life.

CDC. (2018). *Influenza antiviral medications: Summary for clinicians* . https://www.cdc.gov/flu/pdf/professionals/antivirals/antiviral-summary-clinician.pdf.

CDC. (2019a). *Sickle cell fact sheet.* https://www.cdc.gov/ncbddd/sicklecell/documents/factsheet_scicklecell_status.pdf

CDC. (2019b). *Type 2 diabetes.* Centers for Disease Control and Prevention. https://www.cdc.gov/diabetes/basics/type2.html

CDC. (2020a). *Diabetes and pregnancy.* Centers for Disease Control and Prevention. https://www.cdc.gov/pregnancy/diabetes.html

CDC. (2020b). *Gestational diabetes and pregnancy.* Centers for Disease Control and Prevention. https://www.cdc.gov/pregnancy/diabetes-gestational.html

CDC. (2021c). *What is type 1 diabetes?* Centers for Disease Control and Prevention. https://www.cdc.gov/diabetes/basics/what-is-type-1-diabetes.html

CDC (2021d). *High blood pressure during pregnancy.* Center for Disease Control and Prevention. https://www.cdc.gov/bloodpressure/pregnancy.htm

CDC (2021e). *Bacterial vaginosis (BV).* https://www.cdc.gov/std/bv/default.htm

CDC (2021f). *Genital herpes.* https://www.cdc.gov/std/treatment-guidelines/herpes.htm

CDC (2021g). *Primary and secondary syphilis.* https://www.cdc.gov/std/treatment-guidelines/p-and-s-syphilis.htm

CDC (2021h). Urinary tract infection. https://www.cdc.gov/antibiotic-use/uti.html

CDC (2021i) *Sexually transmitted infections treatment guidelines.* https://www.cdc.gov/std/treatment-guidelines/syphilis-pregnancy.htm

CDC (2022a). *Zika.* https://www.cdc.gov/zika/index.html

CDC (2022b). *Pregnant and recently pregnant people at increased risk for severe illness from COVID-19.* https://www.cdc.gov/coronavirus/2019-ncov/need-extra-precautions/pregnant-people.html

CDC (2022c). *STDs during pregnancy- CDC detailed fact sheet.* https://www.cdc.gov/std/pregnancy/stdfact-pregnancy-detailed.htm

CDC (2022d). *Syphilis–CDC Detailed fact sheet.* https://www.cdc.gov/std/syphilis/stdfact syphilis-detailed.htm

CDC (2022e). *Systemic lupus erythematosus* (SLE). Centers for Disease Control and Prevention. https://www.cdc.gov/lupus/facts/detailed.html#sleMakol

Dao, K. H. & Bermas, B. L. (2022). Systemic lupus erythematosus management in pregnancy. *International Journal of Women's Health, 14* (199–211).

Dulay, A. T. (2020a). *Oligohydramnios.* https://www.merckmanuals.com/professional/gynecology-and-obstetrics/abnormalities-of-pregnancy/oligohydramnios

Dulay, A. T. (2020b). *Polyhydramnios.* https://www.merckmanuals.com/professional/gynecology-and-obstetrics/abnormalities-of-pregnancy/polyhydramnios

Hadi, Y. & Kupec, J. (2022). *Fatty liver in pregnancy.* https://www.ncbi.nlm.nih.gov/books/NBK545315

Hsu, K. (2022). *Patient education: Chlamydia (beyond the basics).* https://www.uptodate.com/contents/chlamydia-beyond-the-basics#H1900484613

Kelley, C. E. & Weaver, A. (2019). Diabetes mellitus. *Clinical Updates in Women's Health Care XVIII* (6), 2–32

Krause, M. L. & Makol, A. (2016). Management of rheumatoid arthritis during pregnancy: Challenges and solutions. *Open Access to Rheumatology 8,* 23–36. https://www.ncbi.nlm.nih.gov/pmc/articles/PMC5098768/ doi: 10.2147/OARRR.S85340

Lindley, K. & Williams, D. (2018). Valvular heart disease in pregnancy. *American College of Cardiology.* https://www.acc.org/latest-in-cardiology/articles/2018/02/12/07/29/valvular-heart-disease-in-pregnancy

March of Dimes (2013). *Oligohydramnios.* https://www.marchofdimes.org/complications/oligohydramnios.asp

March of Dimes (2022a). *Scleroderma and pregnancy.* https://www.marchofdimes.org/scleroderma-and-pregnancy.aspx

March of Dimes (2022b). *Sickle Cell Disease and pregnancy.* https://www.marchofdimes.org/complications/sickle-cell-disease-and-pregnancy.aspx

Mitanchez, D., Yzydircizyk, C., & Simeoni, U. (2015). What neonatal complications should the pediatrician be aware of in case of maternal gestational diabetes? *World Journal of Diabetes 6*(5): 734–743. https://doi.org/10.4239/wjd.v6.i5.734

National Institute of Diabetes and Digestive and Kidney Disease (2017). *Type 2 diabetes.* https://www.niddk.nih.gov/health-information/diabetes/overview/what-is-diabetes/type-2-diabetes

National Institute of Diabetes and Digestive and Kidney Disease (2017). *Type 1 diabetes.* https://www.niddk.nih.gov/health-information/diabetes/overview/what-is-diabetes/type-1-diabetes#symptoms

National Heart, Lung, and Blood Institute (2022). *Thalassemia.* https://www.nhlbi.nih.gov/health/thalassemia

Oteng-Ntim, E., Pavord, S., Howard, R., Robinson, S., Oakley, L., Mackillop, L., Pancham, S., Howard, J. (2021). Management of sickle cell disease in pregnancy. A British Society for Haematology guideline. *British Journal of Haematology 194*(6), 980–995. https://doi.org/10.1111/bjh.17671

Pillarisetty, L. S. & Sharma, A. (2022, June). *Pregnancy Intrahepatic Cholestasis.* https://www.ncbi.nlm.nih.gov/books/NBK551503

Preeclampsia.org (2017). *Acute fatty liver of pregnancy can be confused with preeclampsia and HELLP syndrome.* https://www.preeclampsia.org/the-news/health-information/acute-fatty-liver-of-pregnancy-can-be-confused-with-preeclampsia-and-hellp-syndrome

Preeclampsia.org (2021). *HELLP syndrome.* https://www.preeclampsia.org/hellp-syndrome

Simpson, K. R., Creehan, P. A., O'Brien-Abel, N., Roth, C. K., & Rohan, A. J. (2021). *Perinatal nursing* (5th ed.). Wolters Kluwer 392–473.

Slate, C,, Morris. L., Ellison. J., & Syed, A. A. (2017). Nutrition in pregnancy following bariatric surgery. *Nutrients 9* (12), 1338. https://doi.org/10.3390/nu9121338

U.S. National Library of Medicine (2022a). *Disseminated intravascular coagulation (DIC).* https://medlineplus.gov/ency/article/000573.htm

U.S. National Library of Medicine (2022b). *Infant of diabetic mother.* https://medlineplus.gov/ency/article/001597.htm

Vierling, J. M., Stribling, R. J., Herrera, S. Burke, A. E., & Koutrovelis, G. O. (2017). Liver disease: reproductive Considerations. *Clinical Updates in Women's Healthcare, XVI*(1), 2–22.

3 FETAL ASSESSMENT

ANTENATAL TESTING

- A thorough prenatal history can identify risk factors for certain conditions so that monitoring can be done to prevent potential harm to both the pregnant patient and the fetus.
- Antenatal surveillance is now a standard in obstetrics, but no single test has proven to be the definitive test for all situations.
- The goal of antenatal testing is to monitor potential fetal hypoxia or injury and weigh the costs of intervening, especially in very preterm pregnancies.

AMNIOCENTESIS

- This procedure involves the needle aspiration of amniotic fluid and cells to determine genetic abnormalities in the fetus.
- It is performed by passing a long, thin needle through the maternal abdominal wall and the fetal amniotic sac, guided by ultrasound. With a syringe, a small sample of fluid is removed. The fluid sample contains fetal cells.

Gestation Performed

- Amniocentesis is performed during the second trimester, between 15 and 20 weeks for genetic testing.
- It may be performed later in pregnancy to check fetal lung maturity if preterm delivery is anticipated.

Testing Results

- Amniocentesis identifies all fetal chromosomes and detects abnormalities such as missing, altered, misplaced, or additional genetic material.
- It indicates fetal lung maturity by measuring the lecithin-to-sphingomyelin ratio, which should be 2:1 for optimal lung function.
- The normal number of chromosomes is 46.
- Amniocentesis does not test all chromosomal disorders. A negative result does not rule out all genetic abnormalities.

Risks

- Maternal infection
- Miscarriage
- Preterm labor
- Rhesus disease in the fetus if pregnant patient is Rh negative and fetus is Rh positive. If fetal blood cells come into contact with maternal cells during the procedure, the patient can begin producing antibodies, causing rhesus disease in the fetus. RhoGAM should be given following the procedure to prevent this complication.

Reasons for Use

- Amniocentesis does not test all chromosomal disorders. A negative result does not rule out all genetic abnormalities.
- Amniocentesis is done to detect certain chromosomal abnormalities such as cystic fibrosis, Down syndrome (trisomy 21), sickle cell disease, and Tay-Sachs disease.
- Women over 35 are at increased risk of fetal genetic abnormalities.

Patient Education

- The procedure is not painful but may be uncomfortable and cause uterine cramping.
- The procedure takes about 10 minutes, and the nurse monitors you and the fetus for at least 30 minutes following.
- Report any increased cramping or abdominal or vaginal bleeding after the procedure to the provider immediately.

COMPLICATIONS

Genetic screening tests are not required, and all have varying risks. Individual risk factors and family history will guide the choice of genetic study, if any.

CONTRACTION STRESS TEST

- The contraction stress test (CST) is usually done at 36 to 40 weeks.
- The CST identifies the fetal heart rate response to uterine contractions.
- External electronic uterine and fetal heartrate monitoring are applied to the pregnant patient.
- Contractions are induced either by nipple stimulation or intravenous oxytocin, unless contractions are present spontaneously.
- The fetal heart rate is monitored for late or variable decelerations associated with contractions. A contraction pattern of at least three contractions in 10 minutes, lasting 40 seconds or longer, is necessary for adequate testing.
- The CST carries a risk of preterm labor and is contraindicated in the presence of any other risks of preterm delivery or in the case of known placental abnormalities.

Results

- The test is reported as negative, positive, equivocal-suspicious, equivocal, or unsatisfactory.
- **Negative**: the absence of late or variable decelerations
- **Positive**: late decelerations with 50% of contractions
- **Equivocal-suspicious**: intermittent late decelerations or deep variables
- **Equivocal**: decelerations that occur with any contractions more frequent than 2 minutes apart or lasting longer than 90 seconds
- **Unsatisfactory**: fewer than three contractions in 10 minutes or lack of adequate tracing of fetal heart rate or contractions

Risks

- Preterm labor
- Preterm rupture of membranes

Reasons for Use

- The CST is a noninvasive method to screen for potential fetal deoxygenation during labor contractions.
- Variable decelerations could indicate compression of the umbilical cord by the fetus, especially in the case of oligohydramnios. ▶

Reasons for Use (*continued*)
- Late decelerations are indicative of poor uteroplacental oxygen transfer.
- Positive CST is associated with, but not definitive of increased risk of fetal hypoxia in labor, intrauterine growth restriction, or low 5-minute Apgar scores.

Patient Education
- CST has a high false-positive rate. If you receive a positive result, the test will be repeated.
- Recommendations for further testing, treatment, or procedures will be based on how far along you are in pregnancy, along with other considerations.
- Report signs of labor following the test due to induced contractions or any vaginal bleeding.

FETAL GROWTH EVALUATION
- Fetal growth is measured to screen for growth restriction.
- Growth can be restricted due to maternal, fetal, or placental factors.
- The etiology in each case correlates with decreased utero-placental perfusion and decreased fetal nutrition.
- Maternal factors include history of smoking, hypertensive disorders, poor nutrition, and substance use.
- Fetal factors may include congenital heart disease, developmental disorders, and genetic disorders.
- Placental disorders include abnormal cord insertion, abnormal implantation, and placental infarcts.

Gestation Performed
- Fundal height measurements at each visit after 24 weeks
- Ultrasound in second trimester and beyond

Results
- Fundal height measurement normally correlates to weeks of gestation after 24 weeks.
- Growth less than 3 cm of expected is considered restricted.
- Growth restriction is generally determined when the fetus measures in the 10th percentile or less of the expected weight for gestational age.
- **With ultrasound, four measurements are typically included:** abdominal circumference, biparietal diameter, femur length, and head circumference.

Reasons for Use
- The growth-restricted fetus is at risk of associated complications, such as cognitive delay in childhood, hyperbilirubinemia, hypoglycemia, IUFD, and respiratory distress syndrome

Patient Education
- If growth restriction is determined, serial ultrasound assessment will be done every 3 to 4 weeks.
- Routine screening for growth restriction will be done throughout your pregnancy.
- Timing of delivery may be adjusted if the fetus is believed to be at increased risk by delaying delivery.

NONSTRESS TEST
- A reactive nonstress text (NST) is indicative of an absence of fetal acidemia and the presence of a well-developed autonomic nervous system.
- The NST should not be performed prior to 24 weeks because the fetus should not be expected to have a fully developed autonomic nervous system prior to that time.
- The presence FHR accelerations is measured by external fetal monitoring for at least 20 minutes.

Results

- The NST results are referred to as reactive (presence of two FHR accelerations of at least 15 × 15 over a 20-minute period, with or without fetal movement, but if less than 32 weeks, two accelerations of at least 10 × 10 is acceptable) or nonreactive (the fetal heart rate [FHR] does not meet the above criteria). Further testing is required, such as a CST or biophysical profile. If unequivocal after 20 minutes, the test may be repeated for a total of 40 minutes.

Reasons for Use

- Advanced maternal age
- Decreased fetal movement
- Maternal diabetes
- Maternal hypertension
- Maternal thyroid disease
- Multiple gestation
- Oligohydramnios
- Polyhydramnios
- Post-term pregnancy
- Previous fetal demise
- Rh sensitization

Patient Education

- The nurse will use external monitoring to view contractions and FHR.
- The nurse will give you a button to press when you feel fetal movement. This marks the tracing.
- The test should take at least 20 minutes. If the fetus is in a sleep state, the test may be extended until the fetus is awake and more active.
- The use of caffeine, nicotine, sedatives, or other drugs may alter test reliability.
- This is a screening test, and if nonreactive, further testing will be conducted.

PERCUTANEOUS UMBILICAL CORD BLOOD SAMPLING

- Guided by ultrasound, a thin needle is inserted through the abdominal wall into the umbilical vein near the placental insertion site.
- A small sample of blood is collected with a syringe.

Gestation Performed

- After 18 weeks
- During second and third trimester

Results

- Chromosomal analysis identifies genetic abnormalities.
- This direct study of fetal blood cells identifies the presence of anemia, viral infections, and bacterial infections.

Risks

- Bleeding from the cord puncture site
- Infection ▶

Risks (*continued*)
- Premature rupture of membranes
- Transient fetal bradycardia

Reasons for Use
- It gives a faster result than amniocentesis or chorionic villi sampling for viral infections or chromosomal analysis.
- Intrauterine blood transfusion can also be done with the procedure, if needed.
- It may be used with IUGR to measure fetal placental oxygen exchange.

Patient Education
- A sample of blood is taken directly from your umbilical vein with a syringe.
- Risks include infection, bleeding, premature rupture of membranes, premature labor, and fetal demise.
- The procedure is conducted under ultrasound guidance as a thin needle is passed through your abdominal wall, uterus, and amniotic sac.

QUAD SCREEN TEST
- A maternal serum blood test
- **Measures four maternal analytes:** Alpha-feta protein (AFP), dimeric inhibin A (DIA), human gonadotropin (hCG), and unconjugated estriol (uE3)

Gestation Performed
- 15 to 22 weeks

Results
- Test factors in maternal age, presence of gestational diabetes, race, and weight
- Predictive of an individual's risk factors for fetal abnormalities

Reasons for Use
- Calculates risk for open fetal defects, such as spina bifida, trisomy 18, and trisomy 21

BIOPHYSICAL PROFILE
The biophysical profile (BPP) combines the NST with ultrasound to observe four fetal and amniotic fluid components:
- Amniotic fluid volume (presence of a single vertical pocket of fluid greater than two centimeters)
- Fetal breathing movements (one or more episodes of breathing movements of 30 seconds or longer in a 30-minute period)
- Fetal movement (three or more body or limb movements within a 30-minute window)
- Fetal tone (one or more episodes of extension or flexion, or opening and closing of a hand)

Gestation Performed
- Second or third trimester

Results

Each component of the test is given a score of 2 or 0 based on whether the component is present or not present.
- A score of 8 to 10 is considered reassuring.
- A score of 6 is considered equivocal.
- If preterm, the test should be repeated in 12 to 24 hours.
- If term, delivery may be considered.
- A score of less than 4 is considered abnormal, and delivery should be expedited.

Reasons for Use
- It measures the fetal metabolic state via the NST (reactive or nonreactive) and renal perfusion via the amniotic fluid level.
- Oligohydramnios (less than 2 cm vertical pocket of amniotic fluid) correlates with decreased placental function and decreased renal perfusion in the fetus.
- The test may be reported as a "modified BPP" only if the amniotic fluid is measured without the other ultrasound components.
- The presence of a reactive NST and adequate amniotic fluid level is considered normal for the modified BPP.

UMBILICAL ARTERY DOPPLER FLOW STUDIES
- Abnormal flow velocity is correlated with poor placental perfusion, fetal growth restriction, fetal hypoxia, and fetal acidemia.
- The ultrasound waveform of a well-growing fetus shows high velocity end-diastolic flow.
- The waveform in the growth-restricted fetus shows decreased diastolic flow.

Gestation Performed
- Generally, after 24 weeks

Results
- Flow indices measured are systolic velocity (S), end-diastolic frequency shift (D), and mean peak frequency shift over the entire cardiac cycle (A).
- Waveform measurements are reported as pulsatility index (S-D/A), resistance index (S-D/S), and systolic to diastolic ratio (S/D).

Reasons for Use
- It measures vascular resistance and placental blood exchange in the growth-restricted fetus.
- In the case of reduced or reversed diastolic flow, the decision may be made to deliver the fetus prior to term to decrease morbidity and mortality.

> **POP QUIZ 3.1**
>
> Which antenatal test allows for direct examination of fetal blood cells?

GLUCOSE TOLERANCE TEST
- Glucose tolerance test (GTT) measures maternal glucose metabolism over time.
- Baseline fasting blood glucose is obtained first.
- Patient drinks a solution of 50 g to 100 g of oral glucose.

GLUCOSE TOLERANCE TEST (*continued*)

- Glucose level is measured 1 hour later.
- Glucose level may be measured again 2 and 3 hours later.

Gestation Performed

- 24 to 28 weeks

Results

- Cutoff range for 1-hour glucose level is between 130 mg/dL and 140 mg/dL.
- If level exceeds that, the test is generally followed by a 3-hour test.
- **Diagnostic ranges for gestational diabetes are:** Fasting 95 to105 mg/dL, 1-hour 180 to 90 mg/dL, 2-hour 155 to 165 mg/dL, and 3-hour 140 to 145 mg/dL.

Reasons for Use

- Gestational diabetes risks for the fetus are hypoglycemia, intrauterine death, macrosomia, and shoulder dystocia.
- Patients who have gestational diabetes are at greater risk of diabetes and its complications after pregnancy is resolved.

Patient Education

- Your blood will be drawn first for a baseline glucose level.
- You will drink a glucose solution and wait on site for repeat blood draws.
- If screening results are borderline or elevated, further monitoring during pregnancy will be needed.
- If screening results are negative, no further testing is required.
- Do not eat or drink prior to and during testing, including no smoking and no gum chewing.

FETAL MONITORING

FETAL HEART RATE ASSESSMENT

Normal ranges for auscultation are:
- Baseline of 110 to 160 bpm
- Regular rhythm
- Absence of decelerations from the baseline
- Auscultation must be done before, during, and after a contraction to determine the type of deceleration, if present

ELECTRONIC FETAL MONITORING

- Baseline of 110 to 160 bpm
- Moderate variability
- No late or variable decelerations
- Accelerations and decelerations may be present or absent

[ ] **NURSING PEARLS**

For low-risk pregnancies and labor without interventions (e.g., labor induction, epidural), intermittent auscultation may be preferred over electronic monitoring. It allows for more freedom of movement and possibly fewer interventions.

DYSRHYTHMIAS

- Some irregularity in the FHR, such as skipped beats, can be audible, but they are generally benign.
- These skipped or irregular beats typically self-correct in the first hours or days of life.
- True cardiac dysrhythmia is rare and requires expert consultation with maternal-fetal medicine.

Treatment

- Diagnosis of the underlying condition will determine treatment options.

POP QUIZ 3.2

What is the most important predictor of fetal acid–base balance and adequate oxygenation when using electronic fetal monitoring?

TACHYCARDIA

- FHR baseline is greater than 160.
- Tachycardia reflects increased sympathetic or decreased parasympathetic tone.
- Tachycardic dysrhythmias most seen are sinus tachycardia (ST; usually caused by maternal factors such as fever or medications) and supraventricular tachycardia (SVT).
- In SVT, the rate may reach 300 bpm, making it difficult to trace electronically. The monitor may use the autocorrection feature and halve the FHR for traceability. There will be an audible difference in the visual tracing and the actual rate in this case. Treatment will be based on the origination of the rapid rate impulse.

Causes

- **Maternal factors:** fever, infection, dehydration, hyperthyroidism, and use of drugs such as beta-sympathetics, parasympathetics, or cocaine
- **Fetal factors:** anemia, hypovolemia, infection, tachyarrhythmia, and an increased metabolic rate

Treatment

- Treatment of tachycardia begins with determining the cause and taking corrective measures accordingly.
- Notify provider of tachycardia and request a bedside evaluation if accompanied by decreased variability or recurrent late or variable decelerations.
- Tachycardia may be treated with digoxin given to the pregnant patient to control the rate.
- Perform intrauterine resuscitation measures as appropriate.

NURSING PEARLS

When the patient presents with fetal bradycardia, it is essential to determine maternal heart rate simultaneously with the FHR. Fetal demise may be missed if the tracing is of the patient's heart rate rather than that of the fetus.

BRADYCARDIA

- FHR baseline of less than 110 bpm
- May be benign and a normal baseline variation in the fetus

Causes

- **Fetal causes:** cord prolapse, cardiac anomalies, fetal hypoxia, intrauterine growth restriction (IUGR)
- **Maternal causes:** hypoglycemia, hypotension, hypothermia, medications, placental insufficiency, placental abruption, uterine rupture

Treatment

- Treatment of bradycardia begins with determining the cause and taking corrective measures accordingly.
- For cord prolapse, elevate fetal head and expedite delivery.
- Maternal steroids, or a beta-sympathetic such as terbutaline, may be given to increase the FHR.

VARIABILITY

- Variability is an important predictor of fetal acid–base balance and adequate oxygenation at the time it is observed.
- The description of variability depends on visual identification and cannot be determined with auscultation only.
- Variability is present when there are visually apparent fluctuations in FHR from the baseline that are irregular in amplitude and frequency.
- It is obtained by viewing a 10-minute window of tracing with at least 2 minutes of identifiable baseline. The 2 minutes do not have to be consecutive.
- Figures 3.1–3.4 show examples of absent, minimal, moderate, and marked variability tracings. ▶

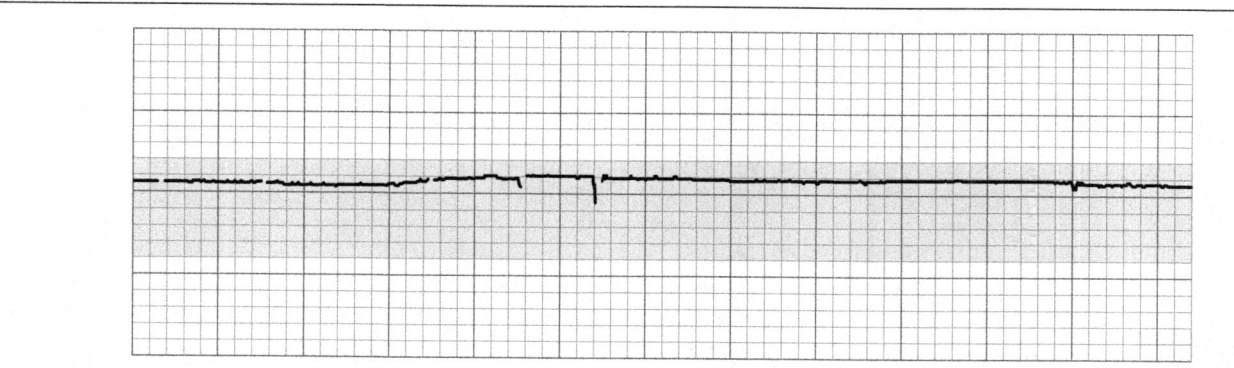

FIGURE 3.1 Absent variability: no visually apparent fluctuations from the baseline.
Source: Nye, R. (2019). *Essentials of fetal heart rate monitoring*. Springer Publishing.

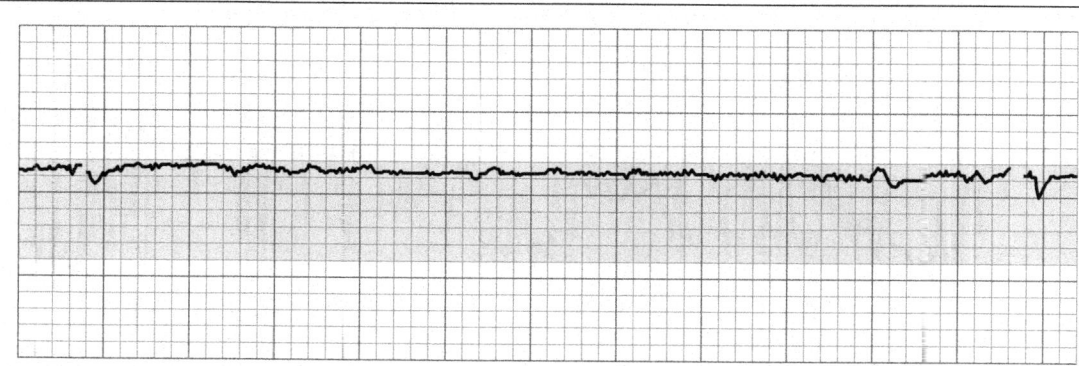

FIGURE 3.2 Minimal variability: visually apparent fluctuations in FHR from the baseline that are detectable, but between 1 and 5 bpm.
Source: Nye, R. (2019). *Essentials of fetal heart rate monitoring*. Springer Publishing.

VARIABILITY (continued)

- **Sinusoidal:** This sign is rare and ominous, appearing as a smooth, sine wave-like pattern with regular undulations that occur 3 to 5 times in 1 minute, and the pattern persists for 20 minutes or longer. It is a sign of a significantly compromised fetus and requires expedited delivery.

ARTIFACT

- The artifact may appear as broken or missing sections of tracing of the FHR.
- It may be due to maternal or fetal movement, poorly attached fetal scalp electrode, poor sound conduction, and/or incorrectly placed ultrasound transducer.

ACCELERATIONS AND DECELERATIONS

Accelerations

- Appropriate central nervous system response to fetal movement ▶

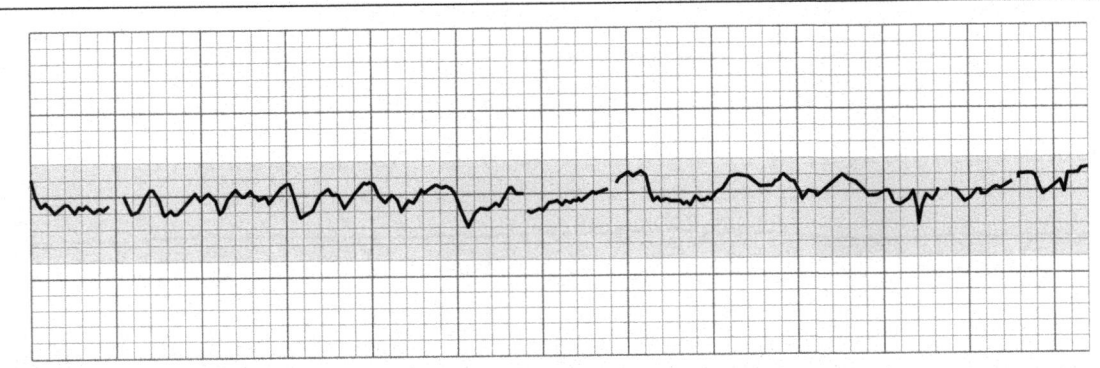

FIGURE 3.3 Moderate variability: visually apparent fluctuations from the baseline that range from 6 to 25 bpm.
Source: Nye, R. (2019). *Essentials of fetal heart rate monitoring.* Springer Publishing..

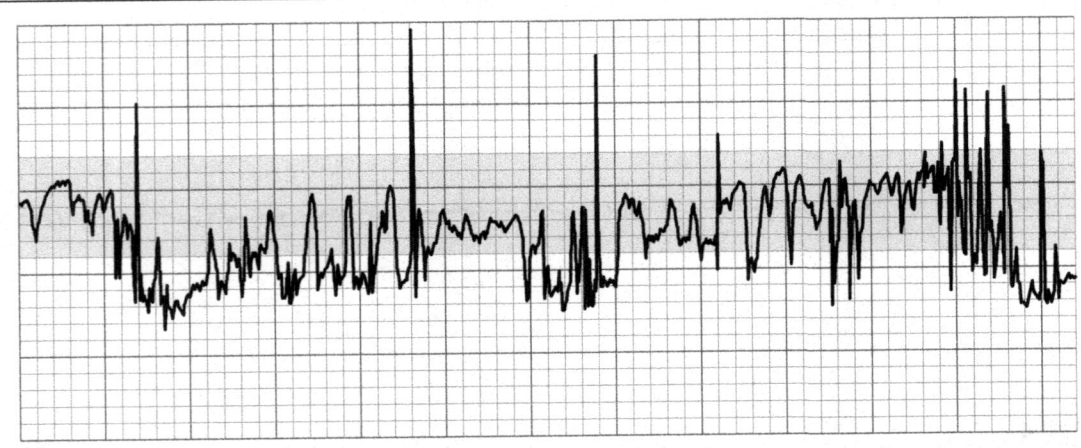

FIGURE 3.4 Marked variability: visually apparent fluctuations from the baseline that are >25 bpm.
Source: Nye, R. (2019). *Essentials of fetal heart rate monitoring.* Springer Publishing.

Accelerations (continued)

- **In the fetus at 24 to 32 weeks of gestation**: An acceleration is an increase from the baseline of at least 10 bpm, lasting at least 10 seconds. They requires a developed central nervous system and therefore are not expected prior to 24 weeks.
- **In a fetus 32 weeks and over**: Accelerations are defined by increases in FHR from the baseline by at least 15 bpm and lasts for at least 15 seconds.
- They can be episodic (occurring with no relation to uterine contractions).
- They can be periodic (occurring with uterine contractions).

Early Decelerations

- They are considered benign and not associated with fetal hypoxia or acidosis.
- They are *gradual* (30 seconds or more from beginning to the lowest point, or nadir) and symmetric in shape, appearing "scooped" from the baseline.
- They coincide with contractions with the beginning, middle, and end of the deceleration mirroring the beginning, middle, and end of the contraction.
- Vagal response caused by compression of the fetal head is the primary cause of early decelerations, and they require no intervention.
- Figure 3.5 shows an example of early deceleration.

Variable Decelerations

- Variable decelerations can be an abrupt decrease in the FHR that is at least 15 bpm below baseline and reaches the nadir in less than 30 seconds
- They can occur with or without relation to uterine contractions.
- Figure 3.6 shows an example of variable decelerations.

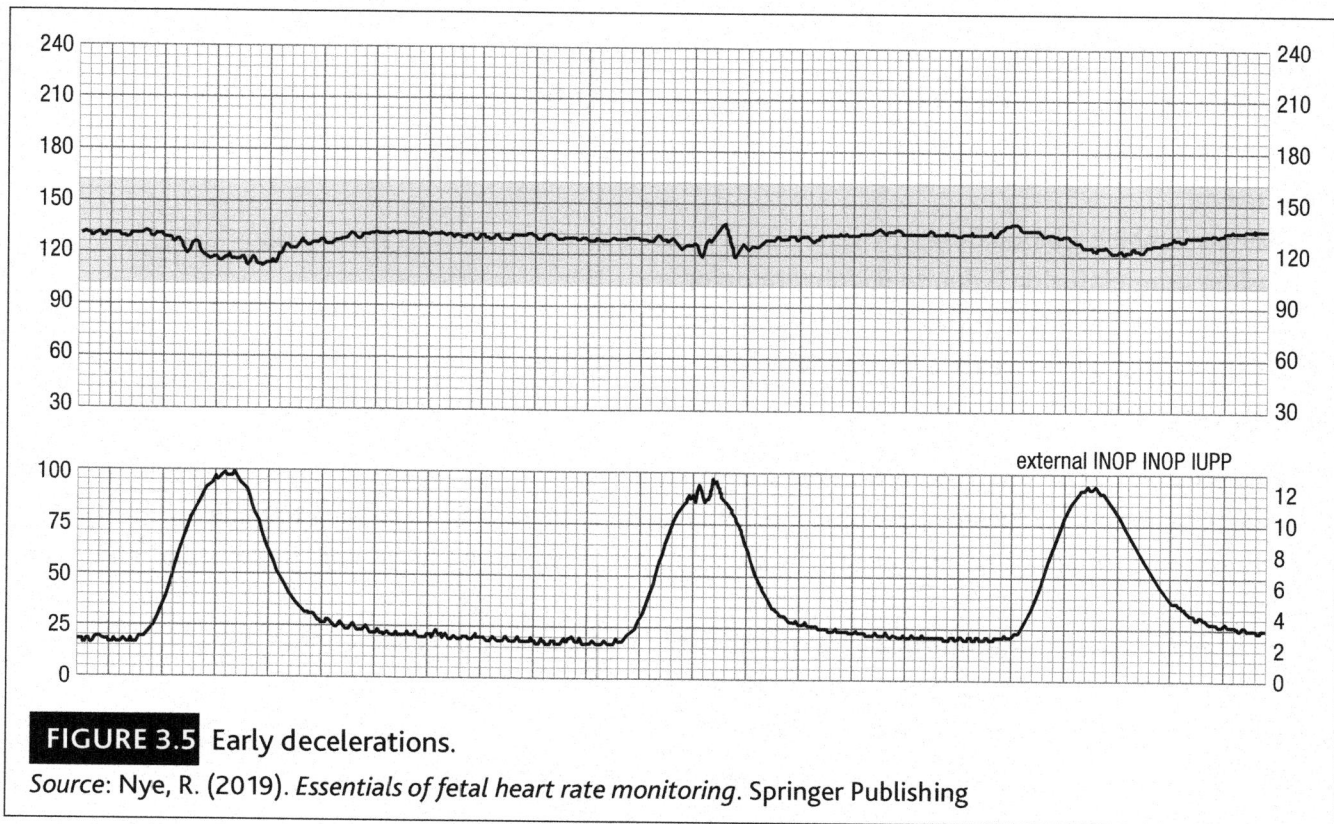

FIGURE 3.5 Early decelerations.

Source: Nye, R. (2019). *Essentials of fetal heart rate monitoring*. Springer Publishing

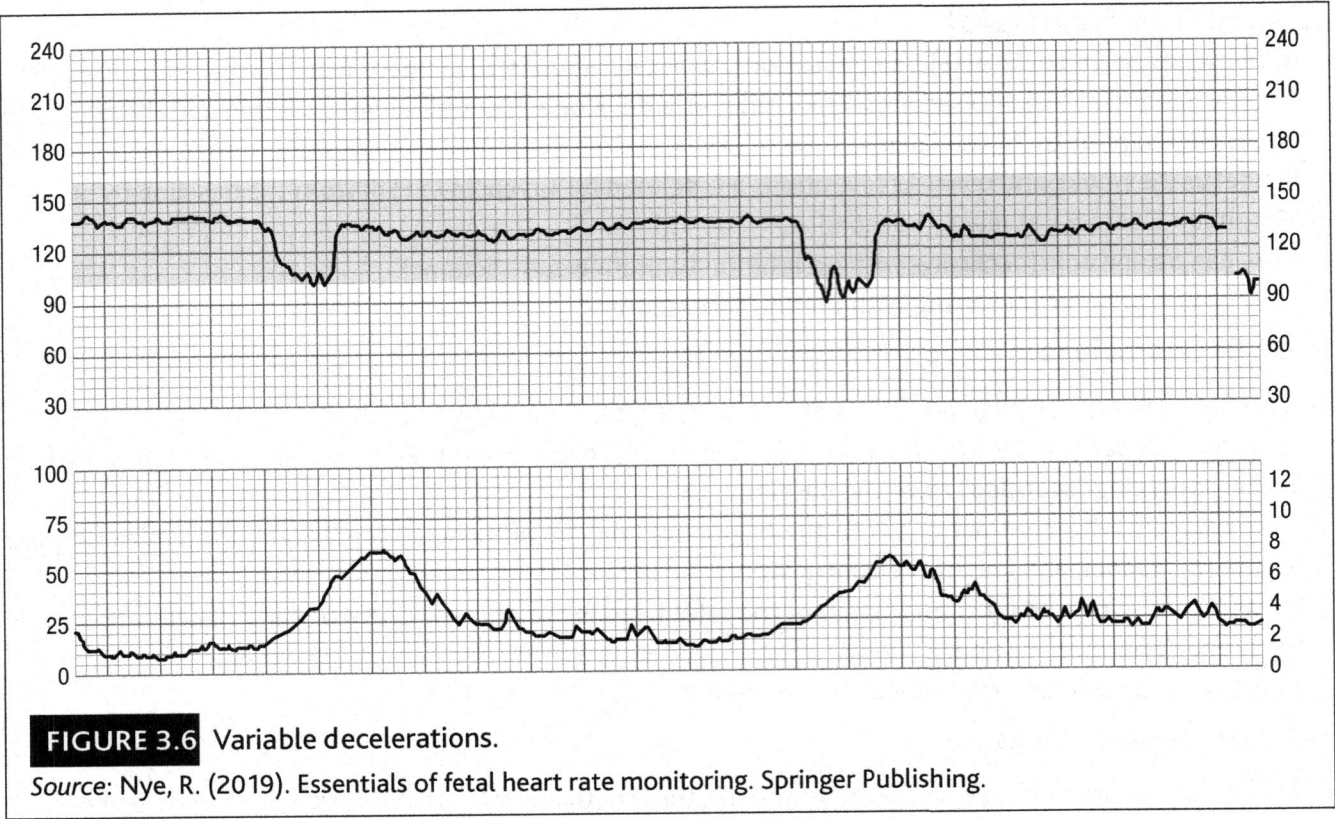

FIGURE 3.6 Variable decelerations.
Source: Nye, R. (2019). Essentials of fetal heart rate monitoring. Springer Publishing.

Causes
- Compression of the umbilical cord, which occludes blood flow to and from the fetus
- Cord prolapse
- Knotted cord
- Nuchal cord
- Oligohydramnios

Treatment
- Maximize umbilical blood flow.
- Consider amnioinfusion if due to oligohydramnios.
- Reposition the patient to move the fetal head off the cord.
- Turn off oxytocin if in use to reduce contractions.

Late Decelerations

- Late decelerations are associated with reduced uteroplacental blood flow.
- *Gradual* decreases in FHR from the baseline, 30 seconds or more from beginning to nadir
- The beginning, middle, and end of the deceleration occurs after the beginning, middle, and end of the contraction.
- Late decelerations are intermittent if occurring with less than 50% of contractions.
- They are recurrent if occurring with greater than 50% of contractions.
- Figure 3.7 shows an example of late deceleration.

Causes

- Insufficient uteroplacental blood flow due to constriction of maternal vessels, defects in cord insertion, infarcts in placental vessels, maternal hypotension, uterine tachysystole

Treatment

- Maximize maternal–fetal blood flow.
- Decrease uterine activity by stopping oxytocin or administering tocolytics.
- Administer maternal fluid bolus of 250 to 500 mL normal saline or lactated Ringers solution.
- Reposition the mother.

Prolonged Decelerations

- Prolonged decelerations are visible decreases from the baseline by at least 15 bpm and last longer than 2 minutes, but less than 10 minutes.
- Any increase or decrease from baseline lasting longer than 10 minutes is a baseline change.
- They may begin as any of the types previously described, but indicate an inability of the fetus to recover from the decreased oxygenation. ▶

[ ] NURSING PEARLS

Remember VEAL CHOP

FHR PATTERN	CAUSED BY
Variable	Cord compression
Early	Head compression
Accelerations	Ok
Late	Placental insufficiency

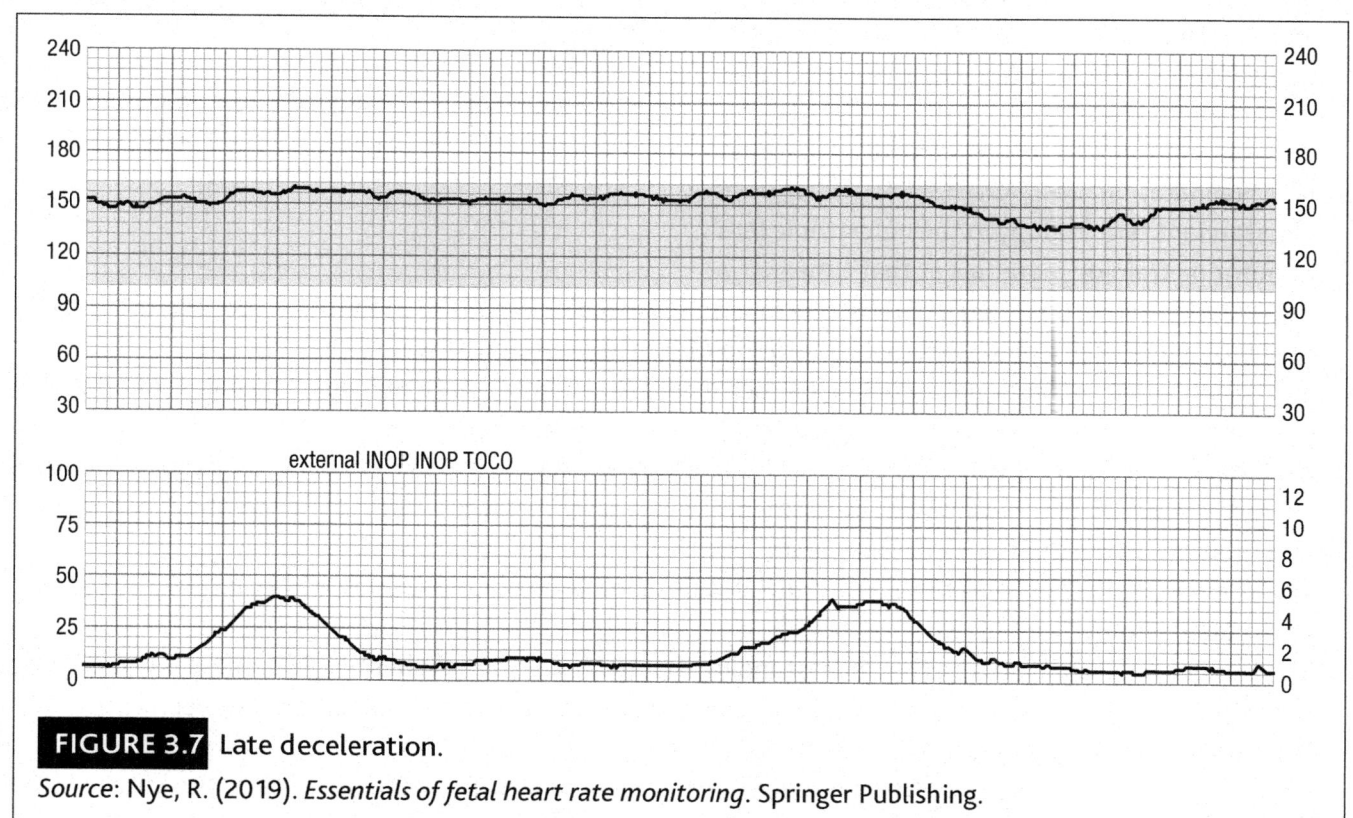

FIGURE 3.7 Late deceleration.

Source: Nye, R. (2019). *Essentials of fetal heart rate monitoring*. Springer Publishing.

Prolonged Decelerations (continued)

- **Early prolonged deceleration**: Gradually begins and ends with the contraction, mirroring the contraction.
- **Late prolonged deceleration**: Gradually begins and ends after the onset and end of the contraction.
- **Variable**: There is a rapid decline from baseline occurring with or without a contraction.
- **Intermittent**: They occur with less than 50% of contractions in a 20-minute window.
- **Recurrent**: They occur with at least 50% of the contractions in a 30-minute window.

Causes
- Sustained instances of cord compression, knotted or shortened cord, head compression, and uteroplacental insufficiency

Treatment
- Correct the suspected cause.
  - Maternal repositioning
  - Fluid bolus
  - Oxygen
  - Amnioinfusion as appropriate
- When paired with minimal or absent variability, or if the prolonged decelerations are recurrent, steps should be taken to expedite delivery.

FETAL HEART RATE CATEGORIES

- In 2008, the National Institute of Child Health and Human Development (NICHD) recommended standardized language to describe fetal heart rate characteristics.
- The Association of Women's Health, Obstetric, and Neonatal Nurses (AWHONN) began using the standard terminology in their electronic fetal monitoring training materials at that time.

 COMPLICATIONS

The category system does not include uterine activity. The full interpretation of the fetal pattern must be evaluated, along with adequate measurement of uterine activity and changes over time, to present the full clinical picture.

- In 2010, the American College of Obstetricians and Gynecologists (ACOG) formally adopted the NICHD terminology as their standard for interpretation of fetal monitoring as well.
- Since then, other professional associations such as the American College of Nurse Midwives (ACNM) and the American Academy of Family Physicians (AAFP) adopted the language.
- When all professionals involved in the care of obstetric patients use the same terminology and descriptive characteristics of the fetal heart assessment, it increases patient safety by decreasing ambiguous communication among the healthcare team.
- The standard of FHR interpretation now includes descriptive characteristics as well as a category system to simplify communication.
- The category system works on the understanding that in labor, normal physiologic processes will change the fetal heart characteristics on a continuum, and we can expect to see movement between categories in relation to those changes.
- With appropriate interventions, the presence of category 2 or 3 tracings can move back into category 1.
- The categories are meant to be a quick and concise way to describe the bedside interpretation to the provider but not limit the full descriptive characteristics charted in the medical record.

Category 1 (Normal)

- The most predictive of a well-oxygenated fetus and a safe uterine contraction pattern

Characteristics
- Baseline between 110 and 160 bpm
- Moderate variability
- Accelerations, present or not
- Early decelerations, present or not
- Absent variable or late decelerations

Interventions
- Continue monitoring for changes.

Category 2 (Indeterminate)

- Interventions must be done, and the provider must be notified of interventions and fetal response.
- This is the most inclusive and most often seen category in labor management. It contains all criteria not included in either category 1 or category 3.

Characteristics
- Bradycardia or tachycardia not accompanied by moderate variability
- Minimal, absent, or marked variability
- Absence of accelerations with fetal movement
- Presence of recurrent variable or late decelerations with minimal, moderate, or absent variability
- Prolonged decelerations
- Absent variability if NOT accompanied by recurrent decelerations

Interventions
- Amnioinfusion
- Assess and treat maternal hypotension
- IV fluid bolus of 500 mL lactated Ringer's solution
- Maternal position change
- Oxygen via nonrebreather at 8 to 10 L
- Pushing with every other or every third contraction
- Reduction of uterine activity if necessary
- Support for maternal pain and coping

Category 3 (Abnormal)

- Indicates a fetus that is hypoxic and in danger of acidosis without intervention
- Requires intrauterine resuscitation and notification of the provider

Characteristics
- Either:
    - Absent variability WITH:
        - Recurrent late decelerations
        - Recurrent variable decelerations
        - Bradycardia
        - Tachycardia
- OR:
    - Sinusoidal pattern

Interventions
- All intrauterine resuscitative measures
- Immediate notification of provider and team
- Preparation for expedited delivery

FETAL SCALP ELECTRODE (FSE)

- Electrode is secured to the fetal head (avoiding the fontanels and face) or the buttocks (avoiding the genitalia).
- It provides more consistent and accurate FHR tracing.
- The direct placement of the electrode measures the R-R wave intervals in the cardiac QRS complex.
- It is used to trace a very active fetus or when ultrasound transmission may be less reliable.
- It is useful if cardiac arrhythmia is suspected.

Contraindications

- Hemophilia
- Herpes infection
- Maternal HIV
- Placenta previa
- Presenting part undetermined

Risks

- In the case of fetal demise, the electrode may pick up the pregnant patient's heart rate signal, and the demise could be missed.
- It is invasive and provides a direct vehicle for bacterial or viral infection.
- It may require electronic troubleshooting.
- It relies on skilled placement to be accurate.
- It requires rupture of membranes.
- Potential for fetal injury exists.
- Use with caution in the presence of Group B streptococcal–positive patients.

UTERINE ACTIVITY ASSESSMENT

- Accurate and complete assessment of fetal wellbeing requires the assessment of uterine activity as well as the FHR.
- Contraction patterns can greatly influence fetal oxygenation and placental function.
- Maternal coping with contractions is also important to consider in the overall maternal–fetal assessment.

Normal Contraction Pattern

- Frequency is assessed in a 10-minute window averaged over 30 minutes.
- Frequency is measured from the beginning of one contraction to the beginning of the next, and duration is measured from the beginning of the contraction to the return to the relaxed state.
- Normal is less than five contractions in 10 minutes.
- The relaxed, or baseline state, of the uterus must be assessed and verified with palpation.

Hypertonic Uterine Contractions

- By palpation, resting tone is described as soft or hard, with hard meaning a nonrelaxed tone.
- Hypertonus is defined as a uterine resting tone above 20 to 25 mm Hg.
- The direct measurement of resting tone can be obtained only by using an intrauterine pressure catheter (IUPC).

Risks

- Decreased flow of maternal blood through the uterine spiral arteries leading to fetal hypoxia ▶

Risks (continued)
- Placental abruption
- Uterine rupture

Management
- Discontinue or decrease oxytocin if in use.
- Give tocolytics such as terbutaline to reduce uterine tone.
- Use a fluid bolus to reduce uterine activity and intensity.

Hypotonic Uterine Contractions

- The uterus is not contracting at an intensity necessary to bring about cervical change.
- This could be due to cephalopelvic disproportion (CPD), lack of tone in the uterine muscle, and/or fetal malpresentation.

Risks
- Fetal injury if due to CPD or other malposition that impedes progression through the maternal pelvis
- Maternal exhaustion with painful contractions without cervical dilation
- Prolonged labor induction or birth

Management
- Assess fetal position.
- Use oxytocin, if needed, to stimulate the uterus to contract adequately.

Palpation

- Manual palpation of the uterus should always be used when assessing uterine activity in labor.
- It may help to verify hypertonus or hypotonus shown by electronic monitoring.
- Resting tone with palpation is described as soft (relaxed) or hard (not relaxed).
- The intensity of contractions can be estimated only by palpation and is described as mild, moderate, or strong.
- **The subjective reference typically used for intensity by palpation compares the feel of the fundus during a contraction to the feel of one's face:** Mild = tip of the nose; Moderate = chin; Strong = forehead.

TOCO–Electronic Monitoring

- It is based on the principle that the uterine fundus changes shape during contractions.
- The monitor converts the pressure detected by the tocodynamometry (TOCO) into a numerical value displayed on the tracing.
- The TOCO detects uterine tension in the maternal skin over the fundus and should be placed where the contraction is felt strongest.
- This requires palpation for proper placement.
- It is used most frequently in labor as it is noninvasive, allows for maternal positional changes, and is a reliable indicator of contraction frequency.

Intrauterine Pressure Catheter

- A barometric sensor on the tip measures pressure inside the uterus.
- The IUPC has the advantage of accurately measuring the pressure intensity of contractions; measuring uterine resting tone, frequency, and duration of contractions; and providing a route for amnioinfusion.
- The IUPC is placed inside the uterus through the vagina against the uterine wall.

Contraindications
- Placenta previa
- The presence of certain maternal infections (herpes, HIV, hepatitis)

Risks
- Damage or perforation to the uterine wall
- Perforation or abruption of placenta
- Requires rupture of membranes

Montevideo Units
- Montevideo Units (MVUs) are helpful when determining if contractions are adequate for cervical change and to guide decision making during labor induction and the assessment of labor dystocia.
- MVU calculation is done by using baseline values and peaks of contractions represented on the monitor tracing.

 **POP QUIZ 3.3**

The G2P1 patient in labor is a prior Cesarean section due to breech presentation. The patient is undergoing a trial of labor and desires to deliver vaginally. The provider wants to augment labor with oxytocin. What type of uterine monitoring would the nurse expect to use in this case?

- This measurement is used to calculate the intensity of uterine contractions.
- Calculation is the sum of each contraction's peak minus the resting tone in a 10-minute period.
- This is subtracted from the peak of each contraction, and then totaled.
- There are variations in what is considered "adequate" for cervical change, but generally, it is 200 to 280.

INTRAUTERINE RESUSCITATION

- Ideally, the fetus begins labor with a reserve of oxygen sufficient to tolerate the stress of contractions.
- Monitoring of the FHR has shown that certain conditions or events in pregnancy or labor may deplete that reserve more readily.

 NURSING PEARLS

The goal of intrauterine resuscitation is to maximize fetal oxygenation. The methods may be used in combination and do not guarantee the absence of fetal acidemia at birth.

- Nursing intrauterine resuscitation interventions used as standard practice are consistent for any situation in which the FHR tracing could indicate that the fetus is not being adequately oxygenated.
- The priority of interventions is based on the perceived physiologic cause of the change in FHR pattern.
- They may be performed in combination or simultaneously.

Maternal Repositioning
- **Lateral positioning, lateral tilt, knee to chest:** This alleviates cord compression by moving the fetus off the cord, maximizes maternal-fetal blood flow by avoiding compression of the patient's major vessels, and reduces uterine contractions

Fluid Bolus
- Increases maternal blood volume and cardiac output
- Improves uteroplacental blood flow and oxygen delivery to the fetus
- Typically, a 500-mL bolus over 30 minutes given IV to increase perfusion

Oxygen
- Other attempts should be made first to improve fetal oxygenation, including maternal repositioning, reducing contractions, and improving maternal-fetal blood flow.
- Oxygen is delivered by nonrebreather face mask at 8 to 10 L per minute. ▶

Oxygen (continued)

- Oxygen should be considered last due to increased risk of cell damage by oxygen-free radicals.
- Oxygen should be used for short periods of time.

Tocolytics

- In the case of uterine tachysystole, tocolytics should be administered to reduce uterine activity. Terbutaline, an asthma drug used off-label as a tocolytic, is the first-line treatment. Nifedipine, an oral agent, is sometimes used to decrease uterine activity.

Amnioinfusion

- Assessment of fluid return should be done to prevent polyhydramnios. It may be performed in the case of suspected or confirmed oligohydramnios.
- It is done through an IUPC.
- It increases fluid volume surrounding the fetus to reduce pressure on the umbilical cord.
- Room-temperature or body-temperature lactated Ringer's or normal saline is used. A total of 250 to 500 mL is infused over 20 to 30 minutes.

Risks

- In premature or growth-restricted fetuses, a cold solution can cause fetal bradycardia.
- It requires rupture of membranes.
- Overdistention of the uterus by infusing too much fluid or infusing too rapidly may occur. It must be used with caution.

Contraindications

- Active maternal infection
- Uterine anomalies
- Vaginal bleeding

RESOURCES

The American College of Obstetricians and Gynecologists. (2021a). Antepartum fetal surveillance. *Practice Bulletin,* 229. https://www.acog.org/clinical/clinical-guidance/practice-bulletin/articles/2021/06/antepartum-fetal-surveillance

The American College of Obstetricians and Gynecologists. (2021b). Fetal growth restriction. *ACOG Practice Bulletin,* 227. https://www.acog.org/clinical/clinical-guidance/practice-bulletin/articles/2021/02/fetal-growth-restriction

The American College of Obstetricians and Gynecologists. (2020). Screening for chromosomal abnormalities. *ACOG Practice Bulletin*, 226. https://www.acog.org/clinical/clinical-guidance/practice-bulletin/articles/2020/10/screening-for-fetal-chromosomal-abnormalities

Lyndon, A. and Wisner, K. (2021). *Fetal heart monitoring principles and practices* (6th ed.). Kendall-Hunt Publishing Company.

Murray, M., Huelsmann, G., & Koperski, N. (2019). *Essentials of fetal and uterine monitoring.* Springer Publishing Company.

Nye, R. (2019). Essentials of fetal heart rate monitoring. In *Essentials of fetal heart rate monitoring.* Springer Publishing. doi:10.1891/9780826174246.0006

4 LABOR AND BIRTH

PHYSIOLOGY

- Changes occur in the myometrium and the cervix progresses during labor, ending in the birth of the fetus.
- Changes are set in motion by hormones and brought about by forceful uterine contractions.
- Primary change is softening and dilation of the cervix, which allows passage of the fetus through the birth canal.

MATERNAL PHYSIOLOGY

- Maternal factors that trigger labor include **decrease of progesterone** (allows estrogen to stimulate the contractile response of the uterus), **increase of oxytocin levels** (stimulates contractions), **pressure of presenting fetal part on the cervix** (stimulates release of oxytocin into the bloodstream), and **stretching of uterine muscles** (causes release of prostaglandin).

Uteroplacental Physiology

Fetal circulation:
- Oxygen-rich blood flows from maternal circulation to fetal circulation via the placenta to the umbilical cord.
- The umbilical vein passes the fetal liver and joins the inferior vena cava.
- Most of the oxygenated blood passes through a shunt, the ductus venosus, where it is taken to the inferior vena cava and then enters the right side of the fetal heart.
- Oxygen follows the steps in the maternal–fetal pathway to transfer from the environment, through the maternal body systems and essential organs, to the fetus. There can be interruptions at any step of the pathway, affecting fetal oxygenation (Table 4.1).

PHYSICAL ASSESSMENT

GENERAL ASSESSMENT

- Although general assessment of a laboring patient is usually focused on the abdomen, the vagina, and the progress of labor, a head-to-toe assessment should be completed for all patients to ensure overall health.

Initial and Ongoing

Initial and ongoing obstetric systems assessment should include the following.
- Cardiovascular assessment, including heart auscultation, murmur, capillary refill, color, and perfusion centrally and of extremities
- Gastrointestinal assessment, bowel sound auscultation, and evaluation for last bowel movement, constipation, or diarrhea
- Generalized or localized edema ▶

Initial and Ongoing (continued)
- Genitourinary assessment of ability to urinate without symptoms such as burning or hematuria
- Level of consciousness, orientation, affect, and any neurologic symptoms including headache, blurry vision, and evaluation of reflexes
- Respiratory assessment including any distress and breath sound auscultation
- Risk of falls and skin breakdown per hospital policy

ABDOMINAL ASSESSMENT
- Abdominal assessment of the pregnant patient can reveal important information about the general health of the patient and fetus.

Initial Assessment
- General size and shape of gravid abdomen
- Level of pain, cramping, or contractions
- Obvious scars
- Palpation and performance of Leopold maneuvers
- Presence of fetal movement externally (if noticeable)
- Skin color and temperature
- Systematic assessment of fetal presentation and position

Ongoing Assessment
- Abdomen (soft, not tense, between contractions)
- Changes in color or temperature of skin
- Level of pain
- Palpation of uterine contractions for intensity and abdominal tone during and between contractions

TABLE 4.1 Oxygen Pathway and Possible Interruptions

STEPS FOR OXYGEN TRANSFER FROM ENVIRONMENT TO FETUS	POSSIBLE INTERRUPTIONS AFFECTING FETAL OXYGENATION AT EACH POINT ON THE PATHWAY
1. Environmental conditions	Alteration in normal maternal respirations of 21% oxygenated air
2. Maternal respiratory system	Impaired gas exchange
3. Maternal blood flow	Decreased cardiac output
4. Maternal vasculature	Impaired blood flow
5. Uterus	Uterine contractions or injury
6. Placenta	Disruption of maternal–fetal gas exchange
7. Umbilical cord	Compression or injury
8. Fetus	Fetal response to interruptions in the oxygen pathway includes consequences such as hypoxia and fetal injury

VAGINAL ASSESSMENT

Initial Assessment

- Lesions on internal or external genitalia
- Presence of discharge or leaking fluid, including color, thickness, and amount
- Vaginal bleeding

Ongoing Assessment

- Amount of vaginal bleeding
- Discharge
- Presence of lesions
- Temperature and color of tissue

STAGES OF LABOR

First Stage

Characteristics

- The first stage of labor happens in two phases: early (latent) labor and active labor. Active labor is further divided into the active and transitional phases.
- Typically, early labor is the longest stage of the process.

[ ] **ALERT!**

Once the cervix has reached 6 cm dilation, the patient is considered to be in the active stage of labor. In the active stage, the absence of cervical change for >4 hours in the presence of adequate contractions or >6 hours with inadequate contractions is considered an arrest of labor in the first stage and may warrant clinical interventions.

EARLY LABOR

- The opening of the uterus, called the cervix, starts to thin and open wider, or dilate.
- The cervix opens to 6 cm during early labor.
- Contractions get stronger, last 30 to 60 seconds, and come every 5 to 20 minutes.
- The patient may have a clear or slightly bloody discharge, called "show."
- The patient may experience this phase for up to 20 hours, especially if giving birth for the first time.
- Multiparous patients may complete this phase in 14 hours or less.

ACTIVE LABOR

- Contractions become stronger and longer and are more painful.
- Contractions come closer together, meaning that the patient may not have much time to relax between them.
- The patient may feel pressure in the lower back.
- The cervix starts dilating faster from 6 to 10 cm (complete dilation).
- The fetus starts to move into the birth canal.

TRANSITIONAL PHASE

- Phase occurs from 8 to 10 cm of dilation.
- Bloody show increases.
- Rectal pressure increases.
- Patient often finds it difficult to cope and expresses discouragement and doubt.
- Membranes rupture spontaneously if not already ruptured.
- Patient may experience the urge to push.

Support Interventions
- Ambulation
- Focused breathing, relaxation techniques, massage
- Hydrotherapy
- Listening to relaxing music or engaging in other distractions (e.g., watching TV, playing games)
- Position changes, including birthing ball, rebozo wrap, lunges, squats
- Pharmacologic management of pain including nitrous gas, IV sedation, epidural anesthetic

Nursing Responsibilities
Nursing responsibilities include monitoring and documentation of the following:
- Comfort measures
- Documentation of any maternal medications and evaluation for side effects
- Fetal heart tones and uterine activity
- Intake and output
- Maternal vital signs
- Pain status and the patient's ability to cope with pain
- Positioning

POP QUIZ 4.1

What is the definitive indication that a patient is in labor?

Second Stage

Characteristics
- The patient begins to push to help the fetus move through the birth canal.
- The second stage usually lasts longer for first-time mothers and for those who undergo epidural anesthesia.
- It is possible for this stage to last only minutes.
- The patient may feel pressure on the rectum as the fetus's head moves through the vagina.
- The patient may feel the urge to push, as if having a bowel movement.
- The head crowns.
- The healthcare provider guides the newborn out of the vagina.
- Arrest of the second stage is defined as at least 2 hours of pushing for multiparous patients and at least 3 hours for nulliparous patients.

ALERT!

Arrest of the second stage is defined as at least 2 hours of pushing for multiparous patients and at least 3 hours for nulliparous patients.

Support Interventions
- Encourage multiple positions for pushing if desired by the patient and allowed by the provider.
- Give clear instructions on quality of pushing and repeating provider's instructions.
- Provide a quiet, calm environment.

Nursing Responsibilities
Nursing responsibilities include all of those for the first stage as well as the following:
- Assist provider and call for help with any complications during delivery of infant.
- Assist with initiation of essential newborn care.
- Coach patient to optimize pushing efforts.
- Chart time of delivery of newborn.

Third Stage
Characteristics
- The third stage of labor is described as the period from the delivery of the neonate until the delivery of the placenta. The third stage consists of placental separation and expulsion.
- Blood loss of 300 to 500 mL occurs as a consequence of placental separation.
- Patient may experience mild uterine contractions.
- Patient feels sensation of fullness in vagina as the placenta is expelled.
- The uterus may change shape and develop firm contractions after expulsion.

Support Interventions
- If the patient and infant are both physically stable, support skin-to-skin contact to facilitate bonding and early breastfeeding.
- If needed, coach patient in relaxation and slight pushing effort to assist with delivery of the placenta.
- Involve patient's supportive partner to watch, touch, and interact with the patient and neonate to include them in the bonding process.

Nursing Responsibilities
- Administer prophylactic oxytocin as ordered and other hemorrhage medications as needed.
- Assist provider with primary repair of episiotomy or perineal laceration as indicated.
- Observe for signs of placental separation and retained placenta.

INDUCTION OF LABOR: CONSIDERATIONS

INDICATIONS

Indications for the induction of labor are not absolute but should consider maternal and fetal conditions, gestational age, and cervical status.
- Chorioamnionitis
- Fetal compromise, such as fetal growth restriction, oligohydramnios, and isoimmunization
- Fetal demise
- Gestational hypertension
- Maternal medical conditions, including insulin-dependent diabetes mellitus, renal disease, chronic hypertension
- Placental abruption
- Postterm pregnancy, defined as pregnancy lasting after 42 weeks' gestation
- Preeclampsia or eclampsia
- Premature rupture of membranes

CONTRAINDICATIONS
- Abruption with bleeding
- Active genital herpes infection
- Invasive cervical cancer
- Pelvic structural deformity
- Placenta or vasa previa
- Prior classical uterine incision
- Umbilical cord presentation or prolapse

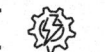 **ALERT!**

Physician and nursing governing bodies have recommended that elective induction before 39 weeks' gestation is contraindicated. Therefore, many facilities will no longer perform elective induction without medical reason until postterm gestation has been reached.

COMPLICATIONS

- Changes in fetal status related to contractions
- Hemorrhage
- Staffing considerations, patient ratios, and patient safety
- Tachysystole
- Uterine infection
- Uterine rupture

BISHOP SCORE

- Cervical status is the most important predictor of successful induction and vaginal delivery.
- Cervical assessment should occur before induction of labor.
- The most common cervical assessment tool is the Bishop pelvic scoring system.
- The perinatal nurse, physician, or provider may perform this assessment.
- **Each of the following factors is scored on a scale of 0, 1, 2, or 3, with 0 being the least favorable for successful induction**: Cervical consistency, cervical dilation, cervical effacement, cervical position, and fetal station are assessed.
- If the total score is greater than 8, the probability of vaginal birth is similar to that of spontaneous labor.

INDUCTION OF LABOR: METHODS

- The following methods may be used to induce labor.

COOK BALLOON AND FOLEY CATHETER

- A single- or double-balloon catheter is inserted by the provider into the extraamniotic space and then inflated with 30 to 80 mL of sterile water to cause direct pressure against the cervix and stretching of the lower uterine segment.
- This is a type of mechanical induction, but it also causes release of local prostaglandins to stimulate labor.
- It may be used in conjunction with pharmacologic methods.
- It may cause significant discomfort in patients with cervical sensitivity.
- The balloon catheter usually falls out with a cervical dilation of 3 cm or more.

AMNIOTOMY

- *Amniotomy* is the artificial rupture of membranes by the provider.
- It is performed with a plastic hook tool created for this task.
- Amniotomy is effective for multiparous patients with favorable cervices.
- Medical record documentation should include indication for amniotomy; amount, color, and odor of amniotic fluid; fetal heart rate characteristics before and after the procedure; and cervical status, including fetal station.

Contraindications

- High fetal station
- Maternal infection such as HIV, active perineal herpes, or viral hepatitis
- Unknown fetal presentation

Risks

- Fetal injury
- Intraamniotic infection
- Umbilical cord prolapse
- Variable deceleration

MECHANICAL METHODS

- There are methods of mechanical induction and cervical ripening other than the transcervical balloon.
- These include membrane stripping and osmotic dilators.

Membrane Stripping

- Digital separation of the chorioamniotic membrane from the wall of the cervix and lower uterine segment by the provider's finger inserted beyond the internal cervical os
- May cause spontaneous rupture of membranes, bleeding, or fever in addition to contractions
- Typically performed in the office at or beyond 39 weeks' gestation

Osmotic Dilators

- Osmotic dilators are medical implements used to dilate the uterine cervix by swelling as they absorb fluid from surrounding tissue. They may be composed of natural or synthetic materials.

Advantages

- Few systemic maternal side effects
- Low cost
- Low risk of tachysystole

Disadvantages

- Maternal discomfort
- Possible disruption of low-lying placenta, causing hemorrhage
- Small increased risk of maternal or neonatal infection

OXYTOCIN INFUSION

- IV oxytocin (Appendix 4.1) exerts a selective action on the smooth musculature of the uterus, particularly toward the end of pregnancy, during labor, and immediately after delivery.
- Oxytocin stimulates rhythmic contractions of the uterus, increases the frequency of existing contractions, and raises the tone of the uterine musculature.
- The physician will place an order for the nurse to initiate. The nurse then titrates per hospital policy, depending on uterine response and evaluation of fetal heart tones.

Nursing Considerations

- Infusion should be discontinued for tachysystole or nonreassuring fetal heart tones.
- Patients should be considered for a 1:1 staffing ratio.
- Patients should be considered high risk for tachysystole. Contractions should be no more than every 2 minutes.
- There may be wide variations in time from initiation of IV oxytocin initial dose to uterine activity.
- Uterine activity and fetal heart rate are continuously monitored and evaluated at 15-minute intervals.

PROSTAGLANDINS

- Prostaglandins (see Appendix 4.1) promote cervical ripening and encourage the onset of labor by acting on cervical collagen and help the cervix to soften and stretch in preparation for childbirth.
- Prostaglandins may also stimulate uterine contractions.
- Most common agents are dinoprostone and misoprostol.

Dinoprostone

- Dinoprostone is administered as a vaginal insert with a removal cord.
- Continuous monitoring of fetal heart rate and contractions is indicated.
- Insert is easy to remove; a speculum exam is not necessary.
- Oxytocin administration should be delayed for at least 30 minutes after removal of insert.
- Patient should remain supine for 2 hours after insertion.
- Uterine contractions usually occur within 5 to 7 hours.

Misoprostol

- Misoprostol can be placed into the posterior vaginal fornix or given orally.
- Continuous monitoring of fetal heart rate and contractions is indicated.
- Oxytocin administration should be delayed for at least 4 hours from the last dose.
- There may be a wide variation in the time of onset of uterine contractions.
- Misoprostol is contraindicated for patients with a history of prior Cesarean section or a uterine scar.
- This drug is inexpensive.

PAIN MANAGEMENT AND COPING

- Most pain during labor and childbirth results from normal physiologic events.
- Pain during labor may result in anxiety and stress, which may have adverse effects on the progress of labor and the well-being of the patient and fetus.
- Addressing labor pain should be a focus of the perinatal nurse.

NONPHARMACOLOGIC METHODS

- Nonpharmacologic methods can include the following.

BIRTHING AND PEANUT BALLS

- Birthing balls and peanut balls may provide physical support and position changes that encourage opening of the pelvis.
- Balls should be used carefully by patients with hip concerns.
- Various positions may be used to help the patient get into a more comfortable position and keep legs and pelvis open to encourage fetal descent.

COACHING

- Coaching consists of emotional labor support such as companionship, eye contact, encouragement, and reassurance.
- Suggestions for new positions or pain relief measures by the coach may help during labor because the patient may not be able to make independent decisions on how to cope during each stage.

HYDROTHERAPY

- Hydrotherapy is considered a cutaneous method of pain relief that reduces painful stimuli.

Benefits

- May decrease use of pharmacologic pain measures
- Enhances fetal rotation due to increased buoyancy
- Faster cervical dilation
- Pain and anxiety relief

Considerations

- Hydrotherapy is safe for use by patients with ruptured membranes.
- Warm water may increase maternal and fetal temperature.
- Watch for maternal dizziness or hypotension.

POSITIONING

- Changing position alters the relationship of the fetus and pelvis, encouraging fetal descent.
- Positioning is a cutaneous method of pain relief.
- Upright positioning increases uterine blood flow and decreases pain.
- Nurses should encourage movement and frequent changes in position during labor.
- Common labor positions include learning forward, rocking in chair, side lying (may use peanut ball, sitting upright, slow dancing with partner, squatting with or without support, standing, and walking.

RELAXATION AND GUIDED IMAGERY

- Relaxation and guided imagery are cognitive techniques that may alter pain perception. The goal is to keep the patient focused and calm.
- The nurse may promote relaxation and a relaxed environment by controlling the amount of noise and interruptions in the patient room; maintaining eye contact (unless it makes the patient uncomfortable); maintaining an unhurried demeanor; sitting next to the patient during assessment instead of standing over the patient; using a soft, calm voice; and using touch or massage if acceptable to patient.
- Guided imagery is a type of relaxation technique that directs thoughts toward pleasant scenes, memories, or experiences. This is often taught prenatally, but the perinatal nurse may encourage use of imagery by guiding patients through imagery.
- Common visualizations include thinking of the baby moving through the birth canal, envisioning the cervix opening like a flower, or simply imagining being on a beach or sitting in the sunshine.

PHARMACOLOGIC METHODS

- Pharmacologic methods include narcotics and nitrous oxide.
- Sedatives are not commonly administered to a patient in labor.

NARCOTICS

- Narcotics (Appendix 4.2) are generally given via IV push.
- Systemic analgesics, otherwise known as opioids or narcotics, reduce awareness of pain and have a calming effect. ▶

NARCOTICS (continued)

- These include butorphanol, fentanyl, nalbuphine, and morphine.
- Because opioids can affect the neonate's breathing and heart rate for a short time, they are often not used within the last hour of delivery.

Side Effects

- Drowsiness
- Itching
- Nausea and vomiting
- Trouble concentrating

> **ALERT!**
> Fetal heart tones may demonstrate decreased variability during maternal narcotic use.

NITROUS OXIDE

- Nitrous oxide (see Appendix 4.2) is a tasteless and odorless gas used as a labor analgesic by some hospitals. It reduces anxiety and increases a feeling of well-being so that enduring pain becomes easier.
- Nitrous oxide is mixed with oxygen and inhaled through a mask.
- The patient holds the mask and decides when to inhale.
- Nitrous oxide is most effective when the patient begins inhaling 30 seconds before the start of a contraction.
- Nitrous oxide is safe for the patient and the fetus. Some patients feel dizzy or nauseated while inhaling nitrous oxide, but these sensations go away within a few minutes.

REGIONAL ANESTHESIA

- Regional analgesia and regional anesthesia are used to lessen or block pain below the waist.
- Methods include the epidural block, spinal block, and combined spinal–epidural (CSE) block.
- Medication includes an anesthetic that may be mixed with an opioid analgesic.
- Medication is given as a single shot or via an epidural catheter.

Epidural

- Anesthesia is injected into the epidural space of the spinal cord to numb the nerves leading to the lower half of the body.
- Typically, a small-gauge catheter is placed to allow continuous delivery of medication until after delivery of the neonate and any needed repairs.

Spinal

- A spinal block starts to relieve pain quickly, but it lasts for only an hour or two.
- Commonly used for Cesarean delivery, it has the same side effects and risks as an epidural block.

Combined Epidural and Spinal

- A CSE block has the benefits of a spinal block and an epidural block.
- The spinal part acts quickly to relieve pain.
- The epidural part provides continuous pain relief.
- Lower dosages of medication can be used with a CSE block than with an epidural block for the same level of pain relief. It has the same side effects and risks as an epidural block.

Side Effects

- Fever
- Headache ▶

Side Effects (continued)
- Hypotension
- Itching
- Soreness

Serious Complications

Serious complications with regional anesthesia are very rare and include the following.
- High epidural or spinal affecting ability of patient to breathe
- Infection at the injection site
- Injury to spinal cord or nerves
- Local anesthetic systemic toxicity
- Numbness, tingling, or rapid heartbeat if the anesthetic is injected into a vein instead of a nerve

GENERAL ANESTHESIA

- General anesthesia is used during childbirth only in special situations or emergencies.
- General anesthesia is given through an IV line or through a mask.
- An anesthesiologist and medical team provide complete care for the patient.

Indications
- Back or spine deformity, causing inability to place epidural catheter
- Contraindications for spinal anesthesia such as bleeding disorders, e.g., thrombocytopenia, or elevated intracranial pressure
- No time to set up spinal anesthesia, such as during an emergency delivery

Contraindications
- Absence of an anesthesiologist or the necessary drugs and equipment
- Cardiovascular failure
- Myocardial infarction
- Severe anemia

Fetal Complications
- Decreased level of alertness after delivery
- Respiratory depression necessitating resuscitation

Maternal Complications
- Aspiration pneumonia
- Decreased bonding with the newborn during longer recovery
- Regular side effects such as nausea, vomiting, sore throat, and shivering
- Respiratory depression
- Toxicity

COMPLICATIONS

Local anesthetic systemic toxicity (LAST) is a life-threatening adverse reaction resulting from local anesthetic reaching significant systemic circulating levels. LAST is rare and almost always occurs within minutes of injection of the local anesthetic. Initial signs and symptoms include agitation, confusion, dizziness, drowsiness, tinnitus, perioral numbness, and metallic taste. Without adequate recognition and treatment, these symptoms can progress to seizures, respiratory arrest, or coma. Initial management of LAST should be focused on airway management, circulatory support, and reduction of systemic side effects. Immediate notification of the anesthesiologist and primary provider is imperative.

POP QUIZ 4.2

A patient just received an epidural for pain management of labor. Which vital sign should be critically monitored after epidural administration?

LABOR PROCEDURES

CESAREAN BIRTH

Indications

- Abnormal or nonreassuring fetal status
- Fetal distress
- Abruption with bleeding
- Breech or malpresentation
- Dystocia of labor
- Placenta percreta
- Placenta previa
- Prolapsed cord
- Prior uterine scar
- Uterine rupture
- Previous Cesarean section

There are no true medical contraindications to the Cesarean section, but if the patient refuses the procedure, it is ethically contraindicated.

Neonatal Complications

- Cephalohematoma, skull fracture, intracranial hemorrhage
- Clavicular fracture, brachial plexus injuries
- Respiratory depression from maternal anesthesia
- Skin lacerations, abrasions, abnormal bruising

Maternal Complications

- Adhesions
- Bowel or bladder injury
- Higher risk of placenta previa, accreta, and increta; placental abruption; and uterine rupture in subsequent pregnancy
- Thromboembolic complications (deep vein thrombosis; DVT)
- Uterine infection

Postanesthesia Assessment Care

- Blood pressure (BP), pulse, temperature, oxygen saturation (SpO_2; every 15 min × 2 h).
- Dressing condition
- EKG monitoring
- Fundal height, tone, and location
- Intake and output
- Level of consciousness
- Lochia amount and color
- Sensory and motor function

Other Important Aspects of Surgical Postpartum Care

- Pneumatic compression devices should remain on patient to prevent DVT.
- Patient should be assessed for nausea and pain.
- Patient should be provided oral nutrition and hydration.

Nursing Responsibilities

- A time-out should be performed before the procedure, which would include checks for antibiotic prophylaxis, correct patient identity, correct procedure to be performed, correct site, fire risk assessment for the operating room, and patient allergies.
- **Preoperative verification process:** Count operative instruments, sponges, and needles to prevent retained foreign bodies. If count cannot be performed due to emergency, an abdominal x-ray should be obtained before leaving the operating suite.

VAGINAL BIRTH AFTER CESAREAN

- Trial of labor after Cesarean (TOLAC) is a planned or attempted vaginal birth after Cesarean (VBAC).
- A birth is officially considered a VBAC once the TOLAC results in a vaginal delivery.
- Patients may desire TOLAC to avoid major abdominal surgery and consequent surgical risk.
- If necessary, TOLAC may result in Cesarean birth after Cesarean (CBAC).

Indications

- One or two previous Cesarean sections
- Cesarean section indication not for prolonged second stage
- History of lower transverse incision

Contraindications

- Any contraindication for vaginal delivery, such as placenta previa or malpresentation
- Previous classical or T incision
- Prior uterine rupture or extensive uterine surgery

Complications

- Cesarean section after failed TOLAC
- Death
- Hemorrhage
- Hysterectomy
- Uterine rupture or dehiscence

Nursing Responsibilities

- Anticipation of complications related to uterine rupture, such as sudden category 3 strip or maternal hypotension
- Continuous electronic fetal monitoring

EPISIOTOMY

- The goal of an episiotomy is to increase the opening of the vagina and perineum to assist with speed of delivery of the neonate.

Indications and Contraindications

- Decreased delivery time in cases of fetal distress
- Operative vaginal delivery with forceps or vacuum
- Shoulder dystocia
- Not recommended as it increases the risk of third- and fourth-degree tears

Complications
- Hematoma
- Hemorrhage
- Infection
- Pain during sex
- Swelling
- Tearing into the rectal tissues and anal sphincter muscle, which controls the passing of stool (third- or fourth-degree tear)

Nursing Responsibilities
- Educating patient about signs and symptoms to report for complications
- Emptying patient's bladder before episiotomy if appropriate
- Providing ice packs, sitz bath, and analgesics to patient after the procedure

OPERATIVE VAGINAL DELIVERY
- Operative vaginal delivery consists of possible episiotomy and use of vacuum or forceps to guide the fetal head and hasten delivery of neonate.

Types
- Depending on training of provider and station and position of fetal head, the provider may use either vacuum or forceps to facilitate birth.

Indications
- Complete cervical dilation
- Engaged fetal head
- Immediate or potential fetal compromise
- Prolonged second stage
- Shortening of second stage for maternal benefit in cases of maternal cardiac disease or maternal exhaustion

Contraindications
- Fetal demineralizing or bleeding condition is suspected.
- Fetal head is not engaged.
- Fetal position is unknown.

Neonatal Complications
- Cephalohematomas
- Facial nerve palsy
- Low Apgar score
- Scalp lacerations
- Seizure

Maternal Complications
- Hemorrhage
- Pelvic floor injury
- **Perineal trauma:** vaginal and perineal laceration, extension of episiotomy, hematoma
- Perineal wound infection

Nursing Responsibilities

- Anticipation and treatment of maternal and neonatal complications
- Catheterization of bladder before procedure

LABOR COMPLICATIONS

PROLONGED PREGNANCY

- Prolonged pregnancy is a pregnancy lasting more than 42 weeks.

Risks

- Fetal and infant mortality
- Presence of meconium in the amniotic fluid
- Stillbirth

Management

- Induction of labor

BREECH OR TRANSVERSE PRESENTATION

Vaginal delivery of an infant in breech presentation may have complications.
- Birth asphyxia
- Intracranial hemorrhage
- Neonatal death

External Cephalic Version

- External cephalic version is the manipulation of the fetus to a cephalic presentation through the maternal abdomen.
- Success rate is 40% for primiparous patient, 60% for multiparous patient.

Indications
- More than 36 weeks' gestation with malpresentation
- No contraindications to vaginal delivery
- Reassuring fetal status

Contraindications
- Previous Cesarean section
- Recent antepartum bleeding
- Rupture of membranes
- Uterine abnormalities

Complications
- Maternal or fetal hemorrhage due to placenta abruption or cord injury
- Premature labor
- Premature rupture of membranes
- Return to the breech position after the procedure
- Transient or persistent fetal bradycardia
- Need for emergency Cesarean section

Nursing Responsibilities
- The nurse is responsible for monitoring vital signs, contractions, and fetal heart tones before, during, and after procedure.
- Regional anesthesia may be used before the procedure, so nursing care may include monitoring return to baseline after administration.

SHOULDER DYSTOCIA

- Shoulder dystocia occurs when there is a need for additional obstetric maneuvers when gentle downward traction has failed to affect the delivery of the shoulders.
- There will be a prolonged time between delivery of the head or presenting part and the rest of the body.

Risks
- Fetal macrosomia
- History of prior shoulder dystocia
- Multiparity
- Postterm pregnancy
- Preexisting or gestational diabetes

Management

McRoberts Maneuver
- The McRoberts maneuver is usually the first maneuver initiated.
- The patient's thighs are hyperflexed against the abdomen.
- This position may ease delivery of the shoulder by changing the relationship of the maternal pelvis to the lumbar spine.

Suprapubic Pressure
- Suprapubic pressure can be used in conjunction with McRoberts and is usually performed by the bedside nurse.
- Firm pressure by the fist or palm of hand in a rocking motion may dislodge the impacted anterior shoulder.
- Pressure is generally applied from the posterior side of the infant.

ALERT!
The nurse should never apply fundal pressure during shoulder dystocia. This may further impact the fetal shoulder.

Other Maneuvers
- Deliberate fracture of clavicle
- Episiotomy
- Gaskin all-fours maneuver
- Wood's screw maneuver

Zavanelli Maneuver
- If all other maneuvers fail, the provider may attempt the Zavanelli maneuver.
- The provider places the fetal head back into the vagina and proceeds with Cesarean delivery.

Documentation
- Documentation should include the time of delivery of the presenting part to the time of complete delivery. Avoid duplicate entries from physician and nurse. ▶

Documentation (*continued*)
- Care should be taken to list each maneuver in the order performed in clear language.
- Avoid minute-by-minute accounts.

AMNIOTIC FLUID EMBOLISM
- Not a mechanical embolic phenomenon but likely a biochemical response where exposure to fetal antigens triggers an overwhelming inflammatory response in the patient
- Most likely to occur during labor and delivery or in the immediate postpartum period
- Causes a triad of hypoxia, hypotension, and coagulopathy

Signs and Symptoms
- Altered mental status, such as anxiety or a sense of doom
- Cardiovascular collapse
- Chills
- Disseminated intravascular coagulation with possible bleeding from the uterus, Cesarean incision, or IV sites
- Fetal distress or bradycardia
- Hypotension
- Loss of consciousness
- Pulmonary edema
- Rapid heart rate or disturbances in heart rhythm
- Seizures
- Sudden shortness of breath

Treatment
- Transfusion of packed red blood cells, fresh frozen plasma, and platelets
- Ventilatory and circulatory support with inotropic drugs as needed

Nursing Responsibilities
- Nursing responsibilities include supportive care. Because of the sudden and severe decline of a patient with amniotic fluid embolism, it is likely to necessitate activation of a rapid response or code team.

PROLAPSED UMBILICAL CORD
- Cord prolapse is descent of the umbilical cord into the vagina ahead of the fetal presenting part, resulting in compression of the cord between the presenting part and the maternal pelvis.
- Cord prolapse is an emergency; immediate delivery will be attempted to save the fetus.

Nursing Responsibilities
- Identify cord prolapse.
- Apply constant pressure to the presenting part with a gloved hand in the vagina to take pressure off the cord until delivery is performed.
- Notify the physician and prepare for emergency Cesarean birth.
- Lower the head of the bed and elevate the patient's hips on a pillow or place the patient in the knee-chest position to minimize pressure from the cord.
- Assess cord pulsations constantly. ▶

Nursing Responsibilities (*continued*)
- Gently wrap gauze soaked in sterile normal saline solution around the prolapsed cord.
- If the cervix is fully dilated, the most emergent delivery route may be vaginal. In this case, the provider may encourage the patient to push and assist with the delivery.

PREMATURE RUPTURE OF MEMBRANES
- Premature rupture of membranes occurs when the membranes rupture before 37 weeks' gestation.

Diagnosis
- History and physical examination sufficient for diagnosis in most cases
- **Digital examination**: to be avoided due to infection risk unless delivery appears to be immediate
- **Speculum examination**: fern test of dried vaginal fluid seen under microscope, vaginal pooling, and visualization of amniotic fluid leaking through the cervix
- pH testing
- PAMG-1 protein marker testing
- Ultrasound for amniotic fluid index

Management
- Management depends on gestational age and current risks.
- Expectant management is recommended and usually includes hospital admission with monitoring for abruption, fetal assessment and contraction status, infection, and umbilical cord compression.

Preterm (for Gestational Ages Greater Than Viability Up to 33 Weeks, 6 Days)
- Antenatal (single course) corticosteroids are recommended.
- Expectant management is recommended and usually includes hospital admission.
- If there are maternal or fetal contraindications to expectant management, delivery is recommended.

Late Preterm (34 Weeks, 0 Days, to 36 Weeks, 6 Days)
- Administer single-course corticosteroids.
- Expectant management or immediate delivery is a reasonable option.
- Monitor for chorioamnionitis.
- Screen for group B *Streptococcus* and administer prophylaxis as indicated.

Term (37 Weeks and Beyond)
- Induction is recommended rather than expectant management.
- If there is no spontaneous labor, induce labor.
- Allow adequate time (12 to 18 hours) for latent phase to progress before performing a Cesarean section for failed induction of labor.
- Screen for group B *Streptococcus* and administer prophylaxis as indicated.
- A short period of expectant management may be offered for 6 hours.

PROLONGED RUPTURE OF MEMBRANES
- Prolonged rupture of membranes is defined as rupture of membranes for more than 24 hours.
- Increased risk of maternal and newborn infection occurs with prolonged rupture of membranes.

Management

- Anticipation of augmentation of labor
- Anticipation of increased risk of neonatal sepsis
- Monitoring of patient for contractions, electronic fetal monitoring
- Possible administration of IV antibiotics or antipyretics
- Vital sign monitoring for demonstration of infection, including maternal and fetal tachycardia

CHORIOAMNIONITIS

- Chorioamnionitis is defined as a bacterial infection of the chorion, amnion, and amniotic fluid. This can lead to infections in both the patient and the fetus.
- The fetus often must be delivered as soon as possible.

Signs and Symptoms

- Fever
- Foul-smelling vaginal discharge
- Maternal and fetal tachycardia
- Sweating
- Uterus that is tender to the touch
- Chorioamnionitis does not always cause symptoms

Management

- Management is similar to that of prolonged rupture of membranes. However, if infection is present, administer antibiotics and antipyretics per orders and prepare for delivery via Cesarean section if vaginal delivery is not imminent.

 POP QUIZ 4.3

A patient is being induced because of rupture of membranes that occurred 2 days ago. During the current shift, the nurse notes the following vital signs: temperature 102.2°F (38.9°C), heart rate 122 beats/min, BP 118/76, SpO_2 95%. Upon the physician's request, the nurse performs a sterile vaginal exam, which is 3/80/−2. What should the nurse anticipate?

APPENDIX 4.1 MEDICATIONS FOR INDUCTION OF LABOR

INDICATIONS	MECHANISM OF ACTION	CONTRAINDICATIONS, PRECAUTIONS, AND ADVERSE EFFECTS
Cyclic nonapeptide hormone (oxytocin)		
• Induction of labor	• Stimulates contractions of the uterus • Increases frequency of existing contractions • Raises tone of uterine musculature	• High risk for tachysystole. Contractions should be no more than every 2 minutes. • Infusion should be discontinued for tachysystole or nonreassuring fetal heart tones. • Adverse effects include nausea, vomiting, and water toxicity.

(continued)

APPENDIX 4.1 MEDICATIONS FOR INDUCTION OF LABOR (continued)

INDICATIONS	MECHANISM OF ACTION	CONTRAINDICATIONS, PRECAUTIONS, AND ADVERSE EFFECTS
Prostaglandin analogues (dinoprostone, misoprostol)		
• Induction of labor	• Acts on cervical collagen to promote cervical ripening • May also stimulate uterine contractions	• Contraindicated for patients with known hypersensitivity to prostaglandins • Contraindicated for multiparous patients with six or more full-term pregnancies • Not used in cases of known fetal distress or vaginal bleeding • May not be used concurrently with oxytocin

APPENDIX 4.2 MEDICATIONS FOR PAIN DURING LABOR

INDICATIONS	MECHANISM OF ACTION	CONTRAINDICATIONS, PRECAUTIONS, AND ADVERSE EFFECTS
Narcotic analgesics (fentanyl, butorphanol)		
• Pain	• Binds to opioid receptors to decrease pain and produce a calming effect	• Side effects include drowsiness, itching, nausea and vomiting, trouble concentrating, and respiratory depression. • Medication may affect the neonate's heart rate and respiratory status. Avoid in the last hour before delivery.
Inhalation analgesics (nitrous oxide)		
• Pain	• Partial opioid receptor antagonist to provide pain relief and produce a calming effect • Mixed with oxygen and inhaled via mask	• Side effects include dizziness, nausea and vomiting, claustrophobia from using the mask, and respiratory depression. • Care should be taken to prevent inhalation of the medication by others in the room.

RESOURCES

ACOG. (2010). ACOG Practice Bulletin 116: Management of intrapartum fetal heart rate tracings. *Obstetrics & Gynecology, 116*(5), 1232–1240. https://doi.org/10.1097/AOG.0b013e3182004fa9

ACOG. (2019). Practice Bulletin 205: Vaginal birth after Cesarean delivery. *Obstetrics & Gynecology*.

AWHONN. (2018). Continuous labor support for every woman, position statement. *Journal of Obstetric, Gynecologic, & Neonatal Nursing, 47*(1), 73–74. https://doi.org/10.1016/j.jogn.2017.11.010

AWHONN. (2018). Fetal Heart Monitoring, Position Statement.

AWHONN. (2019). *Nursing care and management of the second stage of labor* (3rd ed.). Evidence based guideline.

Combs, C. A., Montgomery, D. M., Toner, L. E., & Dildy, G. A. (2021). Society for maternal–fetal medicine special statement: Checklist for initial management of amniotic fluid embolism. *American Journal of Obstetrics and Gynecology, 224*(4), B29–B32. https://doi.org/10.1016/j.ajog.2021.01.001

Cunningham, G., Leveno, K., & Bloom, S. (2018). *Williams obstetrics*. McGraw-Hill.

DeCherney, A. H., Roman, A. S., Nathan, L., & Laufer, N. (2019). *Current diagnosis & treatment: Obstetrics & gynecology*. McGraw-Hill.

Gershenson, D. M., Lentz, G. M., Valea, F. A., & Lobo, R. A. (2022). *Comprehensive Gynecology*. Elsevier.

Ladewig, P. W., London, M. L., & Davidson, M. R. (2017). *Contemporary maternal-newborn nursing care*. Pearson.

Landon, M. B., Galan, H. L., Jauniaux, E. R., Driscoll, D. A., Berghella, V., Grobman, W. A., Kilpatrick, S. J., and Cahill, A. G. (2021). *Gabbe's obstetrics: Normal and problem pregnancies* (8th ed.). Elsevier.

Lawrence, R. A., & Lawrence, R. M. (2021). *Breastfeeding: A guide for the medical profession* (9th ed.). Elsevier.

Lockwood, C., Moore, T., Copel, J., Silver, R., & Resnik, R. (2019). *Creasy & Resnik's maternal–fetal medicine principles and practice*, Elsevier.

Lyndon, A. & Wisner, K. (2021). *Fetal heart monitoring principles and practices*. AWHONN, Kendall Hunt.

Miller, L., Miller, D., & Cypher, R. (2022). *Mosby's pocket guide to fetal monitoring: A multidisciplinary approach* (9th ed.). Mosby.

Siegler, Y., Weiner, Z., & Solt, I. (2020). ACOG, Prelabor Rupture of Membranes, Practice Bulletin. 217. *Obstetrics & Gynecology, 136*(5), 1061. https://doi.org/10.1097/AOG.0000000000004142.

Simpson, K. R. (2021). Fetal assessment and safe labor management, *NCC Monograph*.

Simpson, K. R., & Creehan, P. A. (2021). *AWHONN's perinatal nursing* (5th ed.). Wolters Kluwer.

Tappero, E. P., & Honeyfield, M. E. (2019). *Physical assessment of the newborn*. Springer.

Troiano, N. H., Witcher, P. M., & Baird, S. (2019). *High-risk & critical care obstetrics*. Wolters Kluwer.

5 RECOVERY, POSTPARTUM, AND NEWBORN CARE

POSTPARTUM
Overview

- The *postpartum period*, or puerperium, is the 6-week interval from childbirth to the return of the uterus and other organs to the prepregnant state.
- This time frame can be divided further into the immediate postpartum (first 24 hours), early postpartum (1st week), and late postpartum (2nd to 6th weeks) periods.
- Time during the hospital stay must be well-planned to assist in maternal recovery, newborn care, family preparation, and patient education.

POSTPARTUM ASSESSMENTS
PERINEUM

- The perineum has been stretched and thinned to accommodate the newborn. The appearance of the perineum may vary depending on the type and extent of laceration or episiotomy.
- Assess and document for approximation of the wound, discharge/drainage, ecchymosis, edema, hemorrhoids, and varicosities of the labia.

COMPLICATIONS

Hematomas can develop during delivery. Look for changes in vital signs (VS) without significant bleeding, severe pain to one side of the perineum, or extraordinary swelling or bruising of the labia. Patients may also have difficulty urinating or intense rectal pressure. Alert the provider to these findings, as this can be a hemorrhagic emergency.

Treatment

- Application of ice packs to the perineum for 24 to 48 hours can reduce edema.
- Sitz baths boost blood flow to the perineum to speed healing and relieve soreness, burning, and inflammation.
- **Other treatments for pain and discomfort in the perineum include**: analgesics (oral or topical), a high-fiber diet, witch hazel pads, and ice packs.

Patient Education

- Clean the perineum using a peri bottle of warm water after each urination or bowel movement and pat dry.
- Treat pain with pain relievers, ice packs, and sitz baths.
- Wash and wipe front to back.
- Alert your healthcare provider if you notice foul-smelling discharge or if pulling of sutures in perineum is felt.

FUNDAL HEIGHT

- *Involution of the uterus* is the return of the uterus to its prepregnant size and condition.
- The process begins immediately after the expulsion of the placenta.
- The uterus should be assessed for tone and position.
- Fundal massage is indicated if the uterus is not firmly contracted.
- The lower uterine segment should be supported during massage to prevent prolapse or inversion.
- Assessment of fundal height and lochia should be done per hospital protocols.
- Fundal height decreases by one finger breadth per day and returns to prepregnancy size in 9 to 14 days.

[ ]   **ALERT!**

When the fundus is not midline, it is important to assess the fullness of the bladder, as a full bladder can push the fundus to the side and cause increased bleeding. Encourage the patient to void. If unable to do so, catheterization may be necessary.

LOCHIA

- Assess color, amount, and presence of clots.
- Quantitative blood loss (QBL) should be done for the first 2 hours postpartum for accurate assessment of blood loss.
- The patient may have a temporary increase in lochia when getting out of bed, with breastfeeding, or with large amounts of physical activity.

[ ]   **COMPLICATIONS**

If lochia changes from serosa back to rubra, the patient may need to decrease activity. Bleeding that soaks through one pad in an hour or blood clots the size of an egg or larger can be a sign of postpartum hemorrhage at any point during the postpartum period.

Lochia Stages

Lochia goes through changes during the first 2 weeks.
- **Rubra (birth to 3 days):** bright to dark red color, heavy to moderate flow, possible passing of small clots, fleshy odor
- **Serosa (3 to 10 days):** pink or red-brown in color, significant flow decrease, smaller clots less often, fleshy odor
- **Alba (after 10 days):** yellowish-white color, scant amount, no clots, no strong odor

Patient Education

Report any of the following to your healthcare provider.
- Bright red bleeding that fills a pad in 1 hour or less
- Clots larger than an egg
- Foul-smelling discharge
- Feeling dizzy or lightheaded

PAIN ASSESSMENT

- A standardized tool such as the Numerical Rating Scale or FACES scale should be used to discuss pain with the patient.
- Hot packs may be used for uterine cramping or muscle aches. ▶

[ ]   **COMPLICATIONS**

Extreme perineal, uterine, or incisional pain is considered to be abnormal and should be a cause for concern in the postpartum patient.

PAIN ASSESSMENT (continued)

- **The following may also help with pain management**: analgesics per orders (best effect when taking ibuprofen and acetaminophen together), donut cushions, massage, deep breathing and relaxation techniques, topical sprays and pads.

INCISION ASSESSMENT
WOUND VACUUM

- Negative-pressure wound vacuums reduce edema and bacteria, improve blood flow, and encourage the growth of repaired tissue.

Nursing Interventions

- Monitor function and patency of vacuum, tubing, and canister.
- Inspect occlusive dressing to ensure it remains sealed against patient skin.
- Chart output.

Signs of Infection

- See Infection under Postpartum Complications.

Patient Education

- Follow provider instructions regarding wound vacuum.
- The vacuum may stay in place when showering.
- If you no longer feel suction, notify the provider. The vacuum may need to be removed.
- Know that the vacuum will be removed during your next visit to the provider in 7 days.
- Keep the incision clean, dry, and open to air.
- Remove dressing per provider's orders.
- Report signs of fever, foul-smelling discharge or oozing from the wound or incision site, and other signs of infection.

NURSING PEARLS

Staples placed by the provider should be removed 5 to 7 days postoperatively. An extractor made for staple removal should always be used.

COMPLICATIONS

In rare cases, the incision from a Cesarean section may dehisce. The nurse should always check that wound edges are approximated. Conditions that put a patient at risk for decreased wound healing include diabetes mellitus, hypertension, anemia, smoking, and malnutrition.

ALERT!

Because of concerns for mixing of maternal and fetal blood during delivery, a postpartum dose of Rho(D) immune globulin should be given to Rh-negative patients with Rh-positive newborns. The timing for postpartum dose is as soon as possible after the delivery and within 72 hours maximum.

RECOVERY/POSTPARTUM COMPLICATIONS
OVERVIEW

- Patients in the postpartum recovery period may experience medical complications related to the physiologic changes associated with the reversal from the pregnant state to the prepregnant state.
- During the postpartum period, it is important to associate pregnancy with these complications and look for postpartum-specific attributes of disease processes.

CARDIOMYOPATHY

- *Peripartum cardiomyopathy* is a weakness of the heart muscle that begins sometime during the final month of pregnancy through about 5 months after delivery, without any other known cause. Most commonly, it occurs immediately after delivery.
- It is a rare condition.
- Diagnosis is by exclusion.

Signs and Symptoms

- **Mild:** fatigue, shortness of breath, swelling in lower extremities
- **Severe:** chest pain, extreme shortness of breath, heart murmur, persistence of swelling to lower extremities well after delivery

Treatment

- Prevention of accumulation of fluid in the lungs
- **Medications (see** Appendix 5.1**):** angiotensin-converting enzyme (ACE) inhibitors, beta-blockers, diuretics

Nursing Interventions

- Assess VS and work of breathing.
- Administer supplemental oxygen as needed (PRN).
- Elevate the head of bed to improve lung expansion.
- Monitor for decreasing peripheral tissue perfusion.

COMPLICATIONS

Any complaints of chest pain or shortness of breath in the pregnant or postpartum patient should be addressed immediately by the nurse.

Patient Education

- Report chest pain or shortness of breath, including shortness of breath with exertion that does not resolve with resting.
- Report excessive swelling.

HEMATOMA

- Patients may develop hematoma in the vagina or vulva, causing blood to accumulate in the tissue.
- This can range from a small, uncomfortable hematoma to an obstetrical hemorrhagic emergency.

Signs and Symptoms

- Changes in VS without significant vaginal bleeding
- Severe pain to one side of the perineum
- Vulva or labia with extraordinary swelling or bruising
- Intense pain/pressure in the rectum
- Inability to void

Treatment

- Blood product replacement
- Conservative close observation for hemodynamically stable patients
- **Monitoring:** VS, complete blood count (CBC), fibrinogen, prothrombin time (PT), partial thromboplastin time (PTT)
- For unstable patients: surgical intervention such as evacuation of the hematoma or embolization via interventional radiology

Nursing Interventions

- Monitor VS and vaginal bleeding per orders.
- Obtain labs per orders.
- Place two large-bore IVs.

Patient Education

- Keep the wound clean using peri bottle.
- Report pain and swelling of labia, signs of infection, or lightheadedness/dizziness.

LACERATION

- Lacerations may occur to the cervix or vaginal wall.
- They occur when trauma from delivery causes injury to the cervix or vagina.
- They can be caused by pushing before full dilation, by vacuum or forceps-assisted delivery, or by macrosomia. Lacerations may also occur with a precipitous delivery or spontaneously.

 COMPLICATIONS

Lacerations can lead to postpartum hemorrhage. This type of hemorrhage will not improve with uterotonic medications, intrauterine tamponade balloons, or suction devices, as the uterus is not the source of the bleeding.

Treatment

- **Detection**: often found by nurse
- Repair of laceration by the provider
- Blood replacement
- Hydroxyethyl starch (see Appendix 5.1)
- Tranexamic acid (see Appendix 5.1)

Nursing Interventions

- **Order labs**: CBC.
- **Order a coagulation panel including**: D-dimer, fibrinogen, international normalized ratio (INR), PT, PTT.
- Differentiate between a laceration of the cervix or vagina and bleeding caused by uterine atony.
- Assess vaginal packing that may be placed by provider after repair of the laceration.
- Assess VS.

POP QUIZ 5.1

An hour after a patient delivers, the nurse notes a moderate amount of bright red bleeding trickling from the patient's vagina on examination. The patient's fundus is firm, and the bladder is not palpable. The patient complains of lightheadedness. What should the nurse's next steps be?

Patient Education

- Report increases in lochia or clots.
- Report pain and swelling to perineum.
- Report signs of infection.

INFECTIONS

Postpartum infections may include surgical site infections (episiotomy, laceration, incision), endometritis, mastitis, and urinary tract infection (UTI).

Signs and Symptoms
- Abnormal uterine pain differentiated from uterine cramping
- **Changed VS**: May reflect temperature greater than 100.4°F (38°C), tachycardia, and blood pressure less than 90/50; increase of edema, erythema, or pus from the surgical site
- Malodorous lochia
- Red streaks originating from the wound
- Significant increase in pain reported by the patient

Labs
- Blood culture
- CBC
- Cervical, uterine, or wound culture
- Coagulation studies
- Lactate
- Urinalysis (UA) with reflex to culture

Treatment
- Intravenous/oral (IV/PO) antibiotics
- VS evaluation

Nursing Interventions
- Frequently monitor and report VS outside of normal ranges.
- Monitor the site (e.g., breast, incision) for swelling, pus, or erythema.
- Collect lab specimens and deliver antibiotics.

Patient Education
- Keep the wound clean and dry.
- Leave the wound open to air as much as possible.
- Report fever or chills. A fever is considered a temperature greater than 100.4°F (38°C).
- Report foul-smelling discharge, increased pain, swelling, redness, or pus.
- Report pain, redness, or warmth in breasts or excessive nipple soreness.

COMPLICATIONS

Peripartum infection can develop into SIRS. SIRS is defined by the presence of any two of the following.
- Heart rate (HR) greater than 90
- Respiration rate (RR) greater than 20 or partial pressure of CO_2 less than 32 mmHg
- Leucocyte count greater than 12,000 or less than 4000/μL
- Over 10% immature forms or bands
- Temperature under 96.8°F (36°C) or over 100.4°F (38°C)

RETAINED PRODUCTS
- Retained products may be apparent with delivery of a placenta that is not intact.
- It may also be suspected with increased bleeding or boggy uterus, as the placental fragments get in the way of the uterine muscle's ability to contract.

Treatment
- Treatment for retained products may include bedside curettage or standard surgical dilation and curettage.

Nursing Interventions

- Mobilize operating room (OR) team.
- Monitor VS and QBL.
- Prepare patient for the OR.
- Sedate patient via IV during bedside curettage as appropriate.
- Place two large-bore IVs as there is high risk of hemorrhage with retained placenta.

Patient Education

- Report fever (temperature greater than 101.4°F/38°C) or chills.
- Report foul-smelling vaginal discharge or increase in uterine pain.
- Report sudden increase in vaginal discharge, filling a pad in an hour or less, or clots larger than an egg.

[🧠] **COMPLICATIONS**

Postpartum hemorrhage from retained placenta is not limited to the immediate hours after a delivery. It may occur at any stage in the postpartum period.

THROMBOEMBOLIC DEEP VEIN THROMBOSIS

- Venous stasis, particularly during the latter part of pregnancy, contributes to the risk of the formation of blood clots during pregnancy and the postpartum period. The patient is considered to be in a hypercoagulable state.

Signs and Symptoms

- One-sided calf pain
- Swelling of lower extremities
- Redness of calf or lower leg
- Leg that is warm to touch

Diagnosis

Labs
- **D-dimer**: Of limited value

Diagnostic Testing
- Ultrasound

Treatment

- Heparin regimen for immediate treatment

Nursing Interventions
- Assess for signs and symptoms of complications with heparin therapy such as bleeding or skin necrosis.
- Obtain labs per orders to follow INR.
- Implement preventive care, including sequential compression devices (SCDs) or pulse boots for Cesarean section patients and early and frequent ambulation for all postpartum patients.
- Assess for shortness of breath.

Patient Education

- Report redness or swelling of leg that is painful or warm to the touch.
- Report shortness of breath.

[🧠] **COMPLICATIONS**

Deep vein thrombosis (DVT) is most commonly seen in the lower legs, but clots may move from legs into lungs, causing development of a pulmonary embolism (PE). The patient may suddenly complain of pain in the chest or difficulty breathing. PE may be diagnosed with MRI, ultrasound (US), and/or EKG. Any complaints of chest pain or difficulty in the postpartum patient should be reported to the provider immediately.

POSTPARTUM HEMORRHAGE

- A blood loss of greater than or equal to 1000 mL
- Bleeding associated with signs and symptoms of hypovolemia within 24 hours of birth, regardless of delivery route
- Hematocrit decreased by at least 10 points or more
- Postpartum hemorrhage (PPH) caused by uterine atony, trauma, or patient coagulopathies

Risk Assessment

- Active bleeding
- Cesarean birth
- Forceps-assisted birth
- HCT less than 30
- History of previous PPH
- Known coagulopathy or prolonged aPTT
- Large uterine fibroids
- More than four previous vaginal births
- Multiple gestation
- Placenta previa or low-lying placenta
- Platelet count less than 100,000
- Prior Cesarean section or uterine surgery
- Retained placenta
- Suspected chorioamnionitis or temperature greater than 100.4°F (38°C) with unknown source
- Suspected placenta accreta, increta, or percreta
- Vacuum-assisted birth
- In the United States, The Joint Commission recommends the use of their risk-assessment tool to determine maternal hemorrhage risk prior to delivery.

Labs

There are no labs specific to diagnose PPH. However, the following can be helpful in assessing PPH and response to treatment:
- CBC
- **Coagulation panel, including:** D-dimer, fibrinogen, INR, PT, PTT

Treatment

Treatment depends on the etiology of hemorrhage and includes the following.
- Blood product transfusion
- Dilation and curettage
- Factor VIIa
- Hydroxyethyl starch (see Appendix 5.1)
- Hysterectomy ▶

[ ] **ALERT!**

In vaginal delivery, a blood loss of greater than 500 mL is abnormal and should be cause for concern. Notify the provider to investigate this increased blood deficit.

[ ] **COMPLICATIONS**

Postpartum hemorrhage can become severe enough to cause disseminated intravascular coagulation (DIC).

Treatment (*continued*)

- Intrauterine tamponade balloon, such as cervical ripening balloon
- Intrauterine vacuum-induced hemorrhage control devices
- Repair of cervical laceration
- Tranexamic acid (see Appendix 5.1)
- Uterotonic medications (see Appendix 5.1)
- Uterine massage
- Uterine compression sutures
- Uterine artery ligation

Nursing Interventions

- When performing calculation of blood loss, always perform QBL by weighing and measuring physical blood when possible.
- Have a prepared hemorrhage cart that can be brought into a patient's room to prevent staff from needing to leave the patient to obtain care items. Likewise, have a written guideline to advise staff on the frequency of VS and other assessments.
- Activate obstetrics (OB) hemorrhage protocol.
- Administer drugs and collection of labs per orders.
- Apply vigorous fundal massage.
- Encourage emptying of bladder to encourage uterine contractility either by straight catheter or Foley catheter.
- Encourage inspection of vaginal walls, cervix, and uterine cavity by provider.
- Mobilize team/use chain of command.
- Monitor VS every 5 minutes.
- Place two large-bore IVs, if not in place.
- Prepare for transfer of patient to OR.

Patient Education

- Report bright red bleeding that fills one pad in 1 hour or less.
- Report clots larger than an egg.
- Report dizziness or lightheadedness.
- **Understand signs and symptoms of transfusion reaction, including** back pain, dizziness, fever, chills, or feeling cold, itching, and shortness of breath.

MENTAL HEALTH

OVERVIEW

Routine screening of all postpartum patients for anxiety and depression is recommended using a standardized tool, such as the following.
- Edinburgh Postnatal Depression Scale
- Patient Health Questionnaire-9 (PHQ-9)

[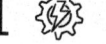] **ALERT!**

The "baby blues" are considered part of normal postpartum adjustment and are defined as a temporary change in emotions after delivery. Symptoms include mood swings, crying, feelings of being overwhelmed, or trouble sleeping. These symptoms resolve between a few days and 2 weeks after childbirth.

Patient Education

For all conditions detailed below, consider the following.
- Join a support group for new parents to help with isolation.
- Report feelings of sadness, hopelessness, or depression lasting longer than a couple of days or affecting daily functioning.
- Sleep when the baby sleeps to achieve maximum rest.

POSTPARTUM ANXIETY

- *Postpartum anxiety* is defined by feelings of dread, constant worry that cannot be eased, sleep disruption, and racing thoughts.
- **Physical symptoms may include** hyperventilation, nausea or vomiting, numbness or tingling of fingers, hands, or mouth, palpitations, and sweating.

Treatment

- Antidepressant medications
- Cognitive therapy
- Complementary therapies such as acupuncture, mindfulness, and meditation
- Exercise
- Sleep health measures

POSTPARTUM DEPRESSION

- *Postpartum depression* is defined by having five or more of the following symptoms lasting longer than 2 weeks after childbirth.
- Screening and treatment for postpartum depression are similar to that for postpartum anxiety and depend on the specific symptoms of the individual patient.

Symptoms

- Decreased or increased appetite
- Diminished ability to think/concentrate or indecisiveness
- Fatigue
- Insomnia or sleeping too much each day
- Marked diminished interest or pleasure in all or almost all activities most of the day
- Psychomotor changes that are noticeable to others, such as slowed movements or agitation
- Sad, empty, or hopeless feelings
- Suicide attempt or recurrent thoughts of death or suicidal ideation
- Feelings of worthlessness or excessive guilt

[COMPLICATIONS]

Suicide or overdose is the leading cause of death for patients in the first year after giving birth. Therefore, it is imperative that the nurse complete depression scoring such as the PHQ-9 on admission to the labor and delivery or postpartum unit.

POSTPARTUM PSYCHOSIS

- Postpartum psychosis usually occurs within the first 2 weeks postpartum.

Symptoms

- Persistent severe insomnia (often present)
- Delusions
- Disorganized behavior
- Hallucinations
- Thought disorganization

Treatment

- Antipsychotic medication (see Appendix 5.1)
- Psychotherapy
- Treatment of insomnia
- Treatment of underlying mental disorder if present
- Sleep when the baby sleeps to achieve maximum rest.

THE NEWBORN

NEONATAL RESUSCITATION

Initial Steps

- The initial steps of neonatal resuscitation include tactile stimulation and drying with warm blankets (can be done on patient's chest).
- During this time, an assessment of the newborn's general state, including a pulse and respiration check, should be completed.
- Place the newborn into the sniffing position.

[⚙] ALERT!

In addition to the labor and delivery nurse, there should be a dedicated Neonatal Resuscitation Program–trained provider at each delivery assigned to the immediate care of the newborn. Consideration of maternal history can be helpful when anticipating the neonate's needs after delivery.

Positive Pressure Ventilation

- If the neonate is apneic or gasping, or if the initial pulse check reveals a pulse of less than 100, positive pressure ventilation (PPV) should be initiated at a pressure of 20 to 30 mmHg and a rate of 40 to 60 breaths per minute.
- If in bed with the patient, the newborn should be moved to a neonatal warmer.
- Listen for rising heart rate during the first 15 seconds of PPV.
- If the HR does not rise and there is no movement of the chest wall during PPV, use corrective techniques to improve the effectiveness of PPV.
- Attach a pulse oximeter to neonate's right wrist or hand.
- Consider cardiac monitoring.
- Use CO_2 detector after advanced airway placement.
- If endotracheal intubation (ET) is performed, continue PPV for 30 seconds after intubation prior to starting compressions.

[⚙] ALERT!

Effective PPV is emphasized because ventilation of newborn lungs is the most effective action in neonatal resuscitation.

Compressions

- After 30 seconds of effective PPV (noted chest rise, positive breath sounds), if the HR remains below 60 seconds, start chest compressions.
- Recheck HR in 60-second intervals.
- Perform cardiac monitoring as the preferred method of assessing the HR during compressions.
- Deliver compressions on the lower third of the sternum to a depth of one-third of the diameter of the chest.
- Use the two-thumb technique.
- Give compressions at a rate of three compressions to one breath.
- Use 100% oxygen to deliver PPV once compressions are started.
- Consider advanced airway any time compressions are needed during resuscitation. If endotracheal tube (ET) intubation is performed, continue PPV for 30 seconds after intubation prior to starting compressions.

Hypovolemia

- If HR persists at less than 60 after 1 minute of compressions, give epinephrine via ET or IV access.
- If indicated by continued persistent low HR and need for resuscitation, or by low blood pressures following a successful resuscitation, administer a fluid bolus of 10 mL/kg of normal saline (NS) or packed red blood cells (PRBC).

Patient Education

- Newborns requiring resuscitation are more likely to be admitted to the neonatal intensive care unit.
- Newborns requiring resuscitation are at risk for sudden unexpected postnatal collapse (SUPC).
- Be vigilant while holding newborn skin-to-skin and during breastfeeding.
- Report changes in color or difficulty breathing immediately to hospital staff.

ADAPTATION TO EXTRAUTERINE LIFE

Overview

- The newborn must adapt from being completely dependent on the maternal patient to being an independent being, a task accomplished over a period of hours to days.
- Successful transition to extrauterine life requires complex interaction between the respiratory, cardiovascular, thermoregulatory, and immunologic systems.
- The following mark the transition from fetal life to extrauterine life.
  - Alveolar fluid clearance
  - Expansion of lungs and decreased pulmonary vascular resistance
  - Circulatory changes, including increased pulmonary perfusion, and the functional closure with change of direction of blood flow in the ductus arteriosus, ductus venosus, and foramen ovale

COMPLICATIONS

Stressors to the neonate, such as hypothermia or hypoglycemia after delivery, may delay or even reverse an infant's transition to extrauterine life. Therefore, it is important to keep the infant warm and dry immediately following birth.

TABLE 5.1 Apgar Score

	0	1	2
Appearance (color)	Blue, pale	Pink body, blue extremities	Pink
Pulse (heart rate)	Absent	Less than 100 beats/min	Greater than 100 beats/min
Grimace (reflex irritability)	Limp	Some flexion	Good flexion
Activity (muscle tone)	Absent	Some motion	Good motion
Respiratory Effort	Absent	Weak cry	Strong cry

INITIAL NEWBORN ASSESSMENT

Apgar Score

- The purpose of the Apgar score is to provide an estimate of how well the newborn is adapting to extrauterine life.
- Assess infant at 1 minute and 5 minutes postdelivery using the Apgar scale (Table 5.1).
- An Apgar score of 4 to 6 indicates a moderately depressed infant, and a score of 3 or less indicates a severely depressed infant.
- Assessment should be repeated at 5-minute intervals if the score remains lower than 7 at the 5-minute score.

Respiratory Effort

- The most important part of the neonate's transition is the onset of ventilation and respiration, which allows newborns to oxygenate themselves instead of relying on maternal circulation for oxygenation.
- Assessment of respirations should occur while the infant is at rest.
- Normal RR is 30 to 60.
- Lung sound should be clear and equal bilaterally.

Abnormal Findings

- **Apnea**: unexplained episode of cessation of breathing for 20 seconds or longer
- **Tachypnea**: respirations greater than 60 breaths/min
- **Grunting**: audible sounds resulting from expired air passing through partially closed glottis as infant increases intrapulmonary pressure to hold alveoli open during respiration; sign of increased work of breathing and respiratory distress
- **Retractions**: depressions observed between the ribs or above or below the sternum that result from noncompliant lungs; sign of distress
- **Nasal flaring**: opening of the nostrils during inspiration as the newborn attempts to open the nasal passage to decrease airway resistance and increase air flow; sign of distress

Normal Vital Signs

- HR: 100 to 160
- RR: 30 to 60
- Axillary temperature: 97.7°F (36.3°C) to 99.5°F (37.5°C)
- Room air oxygen saturation (SpO_2) levels: greater than or equal to 95%

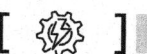 **ALERT!**

SpO_2 levels may depend on altitude. At sea level, it is recommended that SpO_2 remain above 95%. However, at altitudes over 7000 ft, newborns may exhibit SpO_2 levels as low as 90% and be considered to be within normal limits.

Glucose Monitoring

Individual institutions use a range of glucose values; abnormal low values may range from 40 to 55. Glucose monitoring should be performed for newborns at risk of neonatal hypoglycemia.
- Newborns of patients with diabetes
- Newborns of less than 37 weeks gestation
- Newborns with a family history of genetic hypoglycemia
- Large for gestational age (LGA)
- Small for gestational age (SGA)
- intrauterine growth restriction (IUGR)

Newborn Medications

Common prevention medications given to newborns (see Appendix 5.1):
- Vitamin K: IM dose given within 6 hours after birth to prevent hemorrhagic disease of the newborn
- Eye prophylaxis: antibiotic ointment (erythromycin preferred) given in each eye within 6 hours after birth to prevent ophthalmia neonatorum
- Neonatal dose of hepatitis B vaccine: The American Academy of Pediatrics (AAP) recommendation based on research showing greater efficacy when series is started as a newborn

Sudden Unexpected Postnatal Collapse

- SUPC means that a spontaneously breathing newborn at 37 weeks or above gestation with an Apgar score of 8 or greater suddenly becomes limp, pale or cyanotic, bradycardic, unresponsive, and apneic and/or has cardiac or respiratory failure within the first week of life.

Risk Factors
- Category III fetal heart tones (FHT)
- Distraction of caregivers
- Caregiver fatigue
- Newborns requiring resuscitation
- Primiparous mother
- Skin-to-skin contact or breastfeeding with poor positioning

Recommendations
- All newborns in skin-to-skin contact or breastfeeding should be continuously monitored by qualified personnel during the first 2 hours after birth.
- All healthy newborns with risk factors should be frequently assessed during skin-to-skin contact and breastfeeding sessions.
- All caregivers should be taught safe positioning to ensure airway protection and be educated about SUPC and risks such as distraction.

BODY SYSTEMS ASSESSMENT OF THE NEWBORN

SKIN

- The newborn's entire body, including skin folds and scalp, should be inspected and palpated.

Normal Findings

- **Acrocyanosis**: may be seen during neonatal transition, often for the first 24 to 48 hours of life
- **White newborn color**: pink skin tones
- **Newborn with medium skin tones color**: olive or yellow tones ▶

Normal Findings (continued)
- **Black newborn color**: may have reddish-brown tone
- **Erythema toxicum**: normal newborn rash
- **Mild bruising**: may be present from delivery on head, face, or other body parts
- **Milia**: clogged sebaceous glands
- **Dermal melanocytosis**: large, nonblanching lesion over sacrum and flanks, common in Black, Asian, and Native American infants
- **Nevus simplex**: capillary malformations that occur as faint pink patches on eyelids, forehead between the eyebrows, or around the sides of the nose (commonly called "stork bites")
- **Vernix**: odorless, white, protective coating produced by sebaceous glands
- **Lanugo**: fine, soft hair covering the body and limbs
- **Peeling skin**: may be noted in the term or postterm newborn

Abnormal Findings
- **Generalized petechiae**: possible sign of low platelet count
- **Hairy nevi**: type of darkly pigmented birthmark
- **Jaundice occurring within 24 hours of birth**: can indicate liver disease or blood incompatibility issue
- Meconium-stained skin or nails
- Pallor, central cyanosis, or gray skin color
- **Pustules**: could be caused by staphylococcus, streptococcus, or varicella
- **Purpura**: sign of congenital viral infection

COMPLICATIONS
If an infant has meconium-stained skin or nails, the nurse should look for signs or symptoms of meconium aspiration syndrome. These would include cyanosis, increased work of breathing (grunting, flaring, retractions, or tachypnea), or decreased SpO_2 levels. The nurse may also hear crackles or coarse lung sounds upon auscultation of the infant.

Patient Education
- Avoid using baby powder during the first month to prevent inhalation by newborn.
- Bathe newborn every 2 to 3 days. Some providers recommend avoiding the use of a tub until the umbilical stump falls off. Never leave newborn unattended in the tub and gather all supplies ahead of time to have in reach.
- Understand the appearance of newborn rash and other normal lesions to decrease concern.
- Do not peel off dry skin or attempt to remove umbilical stump as this can cause infections.
- Report red streaks, jaundice, or blue or dusky skin.

HEAD AND NECK
Normal Findings
- Ability to move head freely and symmetrically
- Cephalohematoma
- Possible caput, overlapping sutures
- Possible scalp abrasion if fetal scalp electrode (FSE) used
- Head molded if vaginal birth, round if Cesarean birth
- Palpable anterior and posterior fontanels and sutures
- Short neck ▶

Normal Findings (continued)
- Symmetrical head
- Well-formed ears even with or above angle of eye

Abnormal Findings
- Depression of fontanels
- Low-set ears
- Malformations of ear or ear tags
- Multiple nuchal folds
- Palpable fracture of skull
- Subgaleal hemorrhage (notify provider immediately)
- Tension of fontanels or remarkable pulsation of fontanels
- Unusual hair pattern or texture

> **COMPLICATIONS**
>
> The risk of a subgaleal hemorrhage increases with operative delivery such as the vacuum assist. The infant may lose as much as 260 mL blood volume into the subgaleal space. The nurse may feel and see boggy swelling to the head and back of the neck. Bruising may or may not be present.

Patient Education
- Your newborn's hearing will be screened using either the automated auditory brainstem response (AABR) or otoacoustic emission (OAE) test.
- The AABR checks how well the nerve for hearing is working by placing sensors on the newborn's head and neck. When the ears hear a sound, the sensors record the response of the nerve.
- The OAE tests how well the *cochlea,* a part of the ear that detects and responds to sound, is working.

MOUTH
Normal Findings
- Mucous membranes moist and pink
- Tongue of expected size and positioned inside mouth
- Possible neonatal teeth
- Possible Epstein's pearls
- Sucking and rooting reflex noted, possible sucking blisters on lips

Abnormal Findings
- Asymmetry of mouth
- Cleft lip, palate
- Excessive saliva
- Micrognathia or protrusion of tongue
- Persistent circumoral
- Tongue tie/frenulum linguae

Patient Education
- Use a bulb syringe for emesis or buildup of mucus in nares.

> **COMPLICATIONS**
>
> Excessive saliva and respiratory distress during feeding are significant findings. The neonate may be presenting with a tracheoesophageal fistula, a medical emergency.

Patient Education (*continued*)
- Know that feeding can be difficult with cleft lip, cleft palate, or tongue tie. Anticipate referral to occupational therapy, feeding specialists, or surgeons.

EYES AND NOSE
Normal Findings
- Blink reflex
- Mild edema around eyes from delivery
- Patent nares with normal breathing when mouth closed
- Scant amount of clear or white mucus in nares
- Strabismus and/or nystagmus
- Symmetric features with expected placement on face in relation to one another

Abnormal Findings
- Drooping of eyes
- Eyes deviated from center
- Hemorrhage in sclera
- Jaundice of eye
- Nasal flaring
- Nose deviated off center
- Purulent discharge
- Stenosis of nares (choanal atresia)

 COMPLICATIONS

Because infants are obligate nose breathers, choanal atresia can cause cyanosis at rest. When the infant is stimulated for care, they will often pink up as they cry and begin to breathe out of their open mouth. An oral airway can be placed into an infant with suspected choanal atresia to encourage mouth breathing.

Patient Education
- Clear nares or mouth with bulb syringe.
- Report jaundice, or yellowing, of the sclera.
- Report difficulty breathing or excessive stuffiness.

LIMBS
Normal Findings
- Even brachial and femoral pulses bilaterally
- Possible acrocyanosis but similar color/temperature in limbs
- Possible sucking blister on hand or wrist from sucking in utero
- Symmetrical, spontaneous movement of all four extremities, good tone, and flexion

Abnormal Findings
- Asymmetrical movement
- Club foot
- Color difference between extremities
- Crepitus palpated over clavicle or abnormal bump on clavicle
- Webbing of digits or extra digit
- Weakness or absent movement in extremity

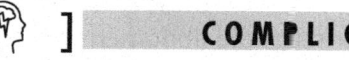 **COMPLICATIONS**

Uneven movement in the infant's upper extremities could be a sign of a brachial plexus injury. This could present as no movement in the newborn's arm or hand or an absent Moro reflex on the affected side. In addition, the infant may extend the arm straight at the elbow and hold it against the body.

CHEST AND CARDIOVASCULAR

Normal Findings

- Capillary refill time of less than 3 seconds
- Equal pulses
- Heart sounds at lower left sternal border (LLSB)
- Intermittent murmur possible during the first few days of life
- Mild irregular breathing from immature central nervous system (CNS)
- Respirations/pulse within normal limits (WNL)
- Symmetrical placement of nipples with breast tissue present in all neonates

Abnormal Findings

- Apnea
- Asymmetry of chest wall or abnormal expansion of lungs
- Asymmetry of nipples
- Bounding or uneven pulses
- Bowel sounds heard in chest
- Heart sounds heard on right side or muffled heart sounds
- Labored breathing, grunting, or retractions
- Persistent murmur

Patient Education

- Report changes in skin color or difficulty breathing.

POP QUIZ 5.2

A low-risk patient delivers a neonate with decreased respiratory effort and cyanosis. The nurse auscultates the newborn's lungs and hears muffled heart sounds and bowel sounds in the chest. The chest is larger than normal, and the infant's abdomen appears flat. What should be the first step in assisting this newborn to ventilate their lungs?

ABDOMEN

Normal Findings

- Three umbilical vessels
- Bluish-white umbilical stump that later becomes dry and brownish black
- Bowel sounds transient or intermittent in the first 24 hours
- Soft, symmetrical, cylindrical contour and relatively prominent abdominal shape

Abnormal Findings

- Abdominal distention or bowel loops
- Abnormal redness, bleeding, or malodorous discharge from umbilicus
- Absence of bowel sounds or hypermobility
- Asymmetrical or scaphoid abdomen
- Bloody stool or emesis
- Gastroschisis
- Omphalocele
- Single umbilical artery
- Umbilical hernia

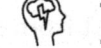

COMPLICATIONS

Green emesis should never be considered normal. This could be a sign of gastrointestinal (GI) obstruction or malformation and should be reported to the provider immediately.

Patient Education

- During diaper changes, fold the diaper down to leave cord open to air.
- Fold diaper away from umbilical cord to prevent irritation and allow it to dry.
- Keep clean and dry; may use mild soap and water daily or with soiling.
- Notify provider for redness, swelling, bleeding, or pus from area.
- The cord typically falls off in 7 to 15 days.

GENITALIA/ANUS
Normal Findings

- Anus patent, in normal position; possible dimpled appearance and infant passing meconium
- Labia majora covering clitoris and labia minora in term infants
- Possible vaginal discharge, including mucus or blood tinge
- Possible vaginal tags
- Swollen labia and scrotum due to maternal hormones
- Testicles descended and palpable in term infants but possibly undescended and palpated in canal
- Urates seen as pink tinge in diapers
- Urethral opening at tip of penis

Abnormal Findings

- Ambiguous genitalia
- Discoloration of scrotum
- Excessive vaginal bleeding
- Hydrocele
- Imperforate anus
- Malformations including epispadias, hypospadias, phimosis, and chordee penis
- Inability to palpate testes

Patient Education

- Avoid using baby powder or talcum powder as the newborn could inhale it.
- Keep one hand on the newborn and have supplies within reach during diaper changes.
- White discharge in female newborn genitalia is a protective layer. Do not attempt to remove.
- Report blood or mucus in stool.
- Know that stools will change from thick, black, and tarry to greenish-black or brown and then transition to runny, seedy, and mustard-yellow.
- Wash hands well with soap and water before and after diaper changes.

POP QUIZ 5.3

The parent of a newborn reports changing multiple diapers containing urine and stool on the newborn's second day of life. During the nurse's head-to-toe exam, the nurse flips the infant over to inspect the spine and buttocks. Upon further inspection, the nurse notes a dimple, but no patent anus. What condition does the nurse suspect?

BACK/SPINE/HIPS
Normal Findings

- Even skin folds on thighs and knees, with even placement
- Lanugo possible over shoulders and back ▶

Normal Findings (*continued*)
- Possible closed pilonidal dimple
- Straight, closed, and easily flexed spine

Abnormal Findings
- Unexpected curvature of spine
- Asymmetric gluteal folds
- Clicking of hips or positive Barlow or Ortolani maneuver
- Malformation of spine, including spina bifida
- Pilonidal cyst or sinus
- Tufts of hair anywhere over spine

COMPLICATIONS
Asymmetry of the gluteal folds could be a sign of developmental dysplasia of the hip in the newborn. The nurse may also note a discrepancy in the length of the legs in the infant. The newborn would require further examination from the provider to check for hip clicking.

NEUROLOGIC
Normal Findings
- Infant easy to console
- Fontanels flat and soft
- Normally pitched, strong cry
- Presence of newborn developmental reflexes
- Tone WNL and symmetrical movement throughout infant's body

Abnormal Findings
- Absent or weak developmental reflexes
- Asymmetrical movement or tone without other explanation
- Infant inconsolable or lethargic
- Persistent fisting
- Tremors
- Seizure
- Weak or high-pitched cry

COMPLICATIONS
Neonatal seizures may present in unusual ways. Some present as stiffening or jerking motions of the limbs or trunk. Other newborns may exhibit cyclical movement of the legs, random or repetitive eye movements, or lip-smacking during seizure.

BEHAVIOR STATES
- Infants may move seamlessly through six sleep/wake states regularly throughout the day.

Deep Sleep
- Smooth and regular breathing
- Few facial movements
- Body nearly still except for occasional startles

Light Sleep
- Some body movement
- Rapid eye movements and fluttering of eyes
- Possible smile or brief fussy sounds
- Irregular breathing

Drowsy

- Mild startles
- Eyes opened or closed
- Eyelids heavy with dull, glazed appearance of eyes
- Some facial movement
- Irregular breathing

Quiet Alert

- Minimal body movement
- Eyes bright and wide
- Face bright
- Most attentive to the environment during this state
- Regular breathing
  - Active alert:
    - Periods of fussiness with much body activity
    - Eyes open
    - More facial movement and increased sensitivity to stimuli
    - Irregular breathing
  - Crying:
    - Increased motor activity
    - Changes in color as infant grimaces
    - Eyes closed tightly or opened
    - Showing limits of comfort reached
    - Irregular breathing

Patient Education

- Report lethargy or difficulty in waking to feed or if newborn will not stay awake long enough for feeds.
- Report unusual fussiness lasting longer than an hour.

NEWBORN COMPLICATIONS

LATE PRETERM INFANTS

- The *late preterm infant* is defined as being between 34 0/7 and 36 6/7 weeks of gestation.
- The infant may initially appear healthy but is at risk of developing many of the problems associated with prematurity.

Signs and Symptoms

Late preterm infants may exhibit:
- Exaggerated jaundice from an immature liver
- Hypoglycemia from low liver glycogen and increased use
- Hypothermia from low brown fat stores
- Increased risk of brain injury
- Poor feeding due to immature sucking reflex and decreased strength of orofacial muscles
- Respiratory distress from decreased surfactant, transient tachypnea (TTN), or pneumonia

Gestational Age
- The new Ballard score tool can be used to determine or confirm gestational age of a newborn. This is most accurate if performed between 10 and 36 hours of age.
- The scoring tool is separated into a neuromuscular assessment and a physical maturity assessment.

Diagnosis
Labs
- Because late preterm infants have an increased risk of hyperbilirubinemia, serial transcutaneous or serum bilirubin testing is recommended starting at 24 hours of age if not sooner, dependent on other risk factors.

Diagnostic Testing
- Early prenatal ultrasonography is a reliable method of determining gestational age.

Treatment
Hyperbilirubinemia
- Phototherapy
- Medical supplementation of feeds
- IV fluids
- Exchange transfusion

Hypoglycemia
- Frequent feedings by breast or bottle
- Glucose monitoring for at least 24 hours after birth
- Glucose gel
- Medical supplementation of feeds
- IV fluids

Hypothermia
- When not skin-to-skin for thermal regulation, the neonate should be dressed and swaddled as much as possible.
- Neonatal warmer with servo-control or an isolette should be used.

Increased Risk of Brain Injury
- No sudden movements
- No laying infant with head lower than rest of body
- No rapid IV boluses if possible

Poor Feeding
- Lactation support
- Medical supplementation
- IV fluids

Respiratory Distress
- Support ranging from nasal cannula to continuous positive airway pressure (CPAP) or intubation
- Administration of surfactant

Nursing Interventions
- Perform car seat challenges prior to infant discharge.
- Increase feeding support, including initiation of pumping of milk for late preterm infants to support milk production.

Nursing Interventions (continued)

- Monitor blood glucose in concordance with hospital orders and policy.
- Monitor vital signs more frequently than in term infants, including pulse oximeter checks and blood pressures.
- Provide additional education to parents regarding risks and management of common late preterm infant (LPI) problems.

Patient Education

- Follow provider's instructions on using supplemental oxygen as needed.
- Know that LPIs may be more difficult to feed. Watch for lethargy or poor feedings, and report them. Report any choking or gagging during bottle feeds.
- Keep infant swaddled and warm; do not unwrap unless absolutely necessary.
- Use phototherapy blankets as needed.
- Report signs and symptoms of hypoglycemia.

[ ] **COMPLICATIONS**

Because of the higher risk for complications in the LPI, staffing ratios should be changed for nurses caring for these infants to reflect their higher acuity.

BRACHIAL PLEXUS INJURY

- *Brachial plexus injury* is defined as the loss of movement or weakness of the arm of the neonate after damage or injury to this group of nerves in the shoulder.
- The nerves of the brachial plexus can be compressed inside the womb or injured during delivery.
- There is an increased risk with breech delivery, infant of diabetic mother (IDM)/LGA infants, and shoulder dystocia.

Signs and Symptoms

- Asymmetrical lack of movement or inability to lift one extremity
- Numbness
- Weakened grip

Diagnosis

Diagnostic Testing

- X-rays
- Nerve conduction study or electromyogram to test nerve or muscle function
- CT scan
- MRI

Treatment

- Most neonates with a brachial plexus injury regain both movement and feeling in the affected arm. In mild cases, this might happen without treatment.
- For a more severe injury, a child will be cared for by a team of specialists from neurology, neurosurgery, occupational therapy, orthopedic surgery, and/or physical therapy
- If pain, weakness, or numbness continues, surgery in the form of nerve or tendon transfer can help.

Nursing Interventions
- Assess neonatal movement and reflexes.
- Coordinate care with adjunct specialties such as physical or occupational therapy.

Patient Education
- Expect a physical therapist to demonstrate specific exercises to do at home to help the newborn improve.
- Massage your neonate as shown by providers.
- Follow up with any recommended providers such as specialists and physical therapists.

LACERATION
- Lacerations on an infant's skin can be caused by scalpels or other instruments during delivery.

Signs and Symptoms
- Most lacerations are superficial and resolve quickly, but some require stitches.
- Wound infection is possible.

Diagnosis
- Visual inspection of wound is all that is required.

Nursing Interventions
- Apply antibiotic ointment or cream to area of laceration.
- Keep wound clean.
- Observe for signs of infection.

Patient Education
- Observe for signs or symptoms of infection.

HYPOGLYCEMIA
- *Hypoglycemia* is blood glucose of less than 40.

Risk Factors
- IDM or gestational diabetes mellitus (GDM)
- LGA
- Late preterm infant
- SGA
- IUGR

Signs and Symptoms
- Apnea or tachypnea
- Cyanosis
- Eye rolling
- High-pitched or excessive crying
- Hypotonia ▶

Signs and Symptoms (*continued*)

- Jitteriness
- Lethargy
- Poor feeds
- Seizure
- Tremors

Diagnosis

Labs

- Glucose check using a glucometer is appropriate.
- Serum neonatal glucose is more specific and should be used for abnormal glucometer values, high-risk neonates, or any time providers need the most accurate results. However, treatment should never be delayed in a hypoglycemic infant while awaiting confirmation of serum glucose.

Treatment

- Dependent on glucose level and presence/severity of symptoms
- Breastfeeding
- Glucose gel
- IV 10% dextrose (D10)
- Supplementation of donor milk, expressed milk, or formula

Nursing Interventions

- Support breastfeeding and lactation.
- Monitor blood glucose.
- Administer glucose gel.
- Insert and care for IV during glucose boluses or infusions if needed.

Patient Education

- Understand why the neonate may be at risk for hypoglycemia.
- Look for and report signs and symptoms of hypoglycemia.

JAUNDICE

- *Neonatal hyperbilirubinemia* is defined as a total serum bilirubin level above 5 mg/dL.

Risk Factors

- ABO or Rh incompatibility
- Asian or Native American ethnicity
- Breastfeeding
- Cephalohematoma or excessive bruising of infant
- Maternal gestational DM
- Significant newborn weight loss
- Male sex
- No stool in first 24 hours
- Prematurity
- Previous sibling with jaundice
- Polycythemia

Signs and Symptoms
- High-pitched cry
- Hypotonia
- Lethargy
- Poor feeding
- Yellowing of skin and eyes

Diagnosis
Labs
- Blood type and Coombs test
- Direct and/or indirect serum bilirubin
- Reticulocyte count
- Serum total neonatal bilirubin
- Transcutaneous bilirubin measurements
- Urinalysis

Diagnostic Testing
- The AAP Guidelines for Phototherapy and BiliCalc App tools are used to determine treatments based on serum level and age in hours of life.

Treatment
- Feeding support
- Phototherapy
- IV fluids
- IV immunoglobulin
- Exchange transfusion

Nursing Interventions
- Breastfeeding and lactation support
- Obtaining blood and urine samples
- Initiation and monitoring of phototherapy
- IV insertion and care during intravenous immune globulin (IVIG) or exchange transfusion

Patient Education
- Report signs of increasing jaundice, such as yellowing of the skin, poor feeding, and lethargy.
- Use phototherapy lights as directed by the provider.

NEWBORN INFECTIONS
- Many microorganisms are responsible for neonatal infection, but group B *Streptococcus* (GBS) and *Escherichia coli* are the most common.

Risk Factors
- Foul-smelling amniotic fluid
- Frequent UTIs
- GBS-positive mother
- Intraamniotic infection
- Maternal sepsis

Risk Factors (continued)
- Preterm labor
- Premature rupture of membranes (PROM)
- Prolonged spontaneous rupture of membranes (ROM)

Signs and Symptoms
- Poor feeds
- Lethargy
- Abnormal VS including unstable temperature
- Hypoglycemia

Diagnosis
Labs
- Blood culture
- CBC including white blood cell (WBC) count
- C-reactive protein (CRP)
- Urinalysis

Diagnostic Testing
- Lumbar puncture to collect and test cerebrospinal fluid (CSF) samples

Treatment
- Antibiotics
- Supportive measures

Nursing Interventions
- Assess and document vital signs.
- Monitor feeding status.
- Assist with drawing labs or lumbar puncture.
- Insert and maintain IV for infants needing antibiotic treatment.

Patient Education
- Report poor feeding or difficulty feeding to the provider.
- Report lethargy or extreme irritability.

[ ] **NURSING PEARLS**

The different pieces of the WBC count provide information on what types of cells the newborn is using to fight potential infection. The following are normal values for a newborn WBC:
- Basophils: 0%–1%.
- Eosinophils: 2%–4%.
- Lymphocytes: 35%–61%.
- Monocytes: 4%–7%.
- Neutrophils: 31%–57%.
- I/T ratio of greater than 0.2 demonstrates infections.
- Absolute neutrophil count may also be used.

NEONATAL ABSTINENCE SYNDROME
- Maternal use of CNS depressants, CNS stimulants, opioids, and hallucinogens are all associated with neonatal abstinence syndrome (NAS).
- Symptoms may start between 24 hours and 10 days after birth and generally last 2 weeks.

Signs and Symptoms
- Fever or unstable temperature
- Overactive reflexes
- Poor feeding and sucking
- Seizures
- Sleep problems ▶

Signs and Symptoms (*continued*)

- Sweating
- Tight muscle tone
- Trembling
- Excessive or high-pitched crying
- Vomiting or diarrhea
- Yawning, stuffy nose, and sneezing

Diagnosis

Diagnostic Testing

- NAS scoring should be done on any newborn of a suspected or known substance user. This is a scoring tool giving numeric value to the signs and symptoms above to detect presence or neonatal withdrawal.

Treatment

- Clustering newborn cares together to allow for longer periods of rest
- Dark room and decreased environmental noise and stimulation
- Decreased tactile stimulation
- Pacifier use
- Small, frequent feeds
- Swaddling and rocking
- Pharmacologic management if symptoms not improved with interventions

Nursing Interventions

- Complete NAS scoring.
- Model appropriate soothing techniques and newborn care to caregivers.
- Reporting of maternal substance use to Child Protective Services (CPS) depending on state statutes.

Patient Education

- Know that newborns with NAS will need to remain in the hospital setting for medical support until they are finished withdrawing.
- Understand that newborns with NAS may be at risk of developmental delay and may need continued outpatient monitoring.
- Understand that involvement with social services may be needed for continued support and observation of the family.

LABORATORY EVALUATION

RH INCOMPATIBILITY

- *Rh incompatibility* is a condition that develops when a pregnant patient has Rh-negative blood and the neonate has Rh-positive blood.
- In a Rh-negative pregnant patient, the immune system treats Rh-positive fetal cells as a foreign substance. The patient's body makes antibodies against fetal blood cells and destroys the neonate's red blood cells.
- Because of the intense red blood cell breakdown, the newborn may suffer from anemia (see below) and jaundice (see above).

Signs and Symptoms

- High-pitched cry
- Hydrops fetalis
- Hypotonia
- Lethargy
- Low or absent blood pressure
- Pallor, then cyanosis and desaturations
- Poor feeding
- Possible normal hemoglobin initially, with rapid decline over 4 to 12 hours with hemodilution
- Shallow, rapid, irregular respirations
- Weak or absent peripheral pulses

Diagnosis

Labs

- Bilirubin testing
- CBC
- Cord (or newborn sample) blood type and screen
- Coombs test

Treatment

- Electrolytes to regulate metabolism
- Hydration
- Phototherapy
- Series of blood transfusions

Prevention is preferred to treatment and consists of $rh_o(D)$ immune globulin at 28 weeks' gestation and with miscarriage or trauma in a pregnant Rh-negative patient.

Nursing Interventions

- Take proper maternal history, including any previous possible miscarriage and timing of $rh_o(D)$ immune globulin injections in the past and during current pregnancy.
- Notify provider for concerns regarding newborn assessment.

Patient Education

- If Rh-negative, understand the importance of $rh_o(D)$ immune globulin during pregnancy for the prevention of Rh incompatibility.

ANEMIA

- Normal hematocrit/hemoglobin (H/H) for term newborn is 18 to 21 g/dL/51% to 68%.
- **Decreased RBC production**: infection, nutritional deficiencies, leukemia, bone marrow failure, anemia of prematurity
- **Increased RBC destruction**: hemolytic anemia, blood incompatibility, infection, other rare diseases
- **Blood loss**: iatrogenic, obstetric accidents, cord/placenta malformation abruption, DIC
- Anemia of prematurity may be an exaggerated physiologic response or be pathologic.
- All infants experience a progressive Hg decline in the 8 to 10 weeks following birth. Anemia is not necessarily symptomatic and is possibly related to rapid body growth, shortened RBC lifespan, and low blood erythropoietin.

Signs and Symptoms

- Low or absent blood pressure
- Pallor, then cyanosis and desaturations
- Possible normal hemoglobin initially, with rapid decline over 4 to 12 hours with hemodilution
- Shallow, rapid, irregular respirations
- Weak or absent peripheral pulses

Diagnosis

Labs

- Bilirubin testing
- CBC
- Coagulation panel
- Cord (or newborn sample) blood type and screen
- Coombs test

Treatment

- Delayed cord clamping
- Limited blood draws
- **Transfusion PRBCs for acute blood loss**: 10 ml/kg
- **If blood unavailable**: saline 10 mL/kg

Nursing Interventions

- Assess signs and symptoms and report to provider.
- Collect labs.
- Monitor problems during blood transfusions.

Patient Education

- Report pallor or shallow, weak respirations.

POLYCYTHEMIA

- *Polycythemia* is an abnormal increase in RBCs, defined as HCT greater or equal to 65%.

Signs and Symptoms

- Apnea
- Cyanosis
- Feeding problems
- Lethargy
- Plethora
- Proteinuria from renal vein thrombosis
- Respiratory distress
- Tachypnea

Diagnosis

Labs

- CBC
- H/H

Treatment

- IV hydration

Nursing Interventions

- Assess signs and symptoms to report to provider.
- Collect labs.

Patient Education

- Understand diagnosis and treatment options.

THROMBOCYTOPENIA

- Normal newborn platelet count is 150,000 to 450,000.
- *Thrombocytopenia* is a deficiency of platelets in the blood.
- Etiologic factors include platelet destruction: maternal autoimmune disorder (e.g., immune thrombocytopenia [ITP], lupus).
- Neonatal conditions
  - DIC
  - Birth asphyxia
  - Infection
  - Large hemangiomas

Signs and Symptoms

- Bleeding from mucous membranes, umbilical cord, or puncture sites
- Cephalohematoma
- Ecchymosis over presenting part
- Petechiae
- Purpura

Diagnosis

Labs
- Blood gases
- CBC
- Coagulation panel
- CRP

Treatment

- Administration of IVIG or platelet transfusion

Nursing Interventions

- Assess signs and symptoms and report to provider.
- Collect labs.

Patient Education

- Understand diagnosis and treatment options.

INFANT NUTRITION

BREASTFEEDING

Breast Changes

- Areola growth in diameter and darkening
- Breast enlargement
- Enlargement of nipples and Montgomery glands
- Internal changes with development of lobules and alveoli of milk ducts
- Skin stretching and appearing thinner with more visible veins

Milk Production

- *Lactogenesis I* begins midpregnancy, with the first stage lasting into the first 2 days postpartum.
- Colostrum may leak from the breasts during pregnancy.
- *Lactogenesis II* is defined as the onset of copious milk production, normally presenting 48 to 72 hours after birth.
- *Lactogenesis III* is defined by the established mature supply of milk.

Hormones

- The two most prevalent hormones of lactation are prolactin and oxytocin.
- **Prolactin**: Levels increase markedly during pregnancy and stimulate growth and development of mammary tissue. Newborn suckling stimulates an increase in prolactin levels, stimulating milk production. Higher prolactin levels at night and nighttime feeding are important to help milk production.
- **Oxytocin**: This hormone helps to contract the cells around the alveoli, which produces ejection and let down. Not only physical in action, oxytocin can create letdown when thinking of or smelling an infant or hearing an infant cry. Frequent contact between mother and newborn encourages an increase in oxytocin.

POP QUIZ 5.4

How would the nurse describe the letdown reflex, including hormone control?

Techniques

- Chest and stomach in line and resting against mother's body (stomach to stomach)
- Chin touching breast
- Flared lips
- Once milk is in, swallowing heard or seen
- Pain free
- Slight movement in jaw up toward ears
- Tongue underneath breast
- Wide gape around breast tissue, not just nipple

Supportive Hospital Practices

- Infant rooming in with patient
- Not giving out gifts or marketing materials provided by formula companies
- No pacifier use during establishment of breastfeeding (with exception of patient request or painful procedure)
- No supplementation without provider order or medical need
- Restricting visitors during the first 2 hours after delivery to encourage skin-to-skin contact and breastfeeding and to prevent SUPC

Contraindications

- Active Ebola infection
- Active untreated tuberculosis
- HIV (in the United States)
- Substance use
- Herpes simplex virus (HSV) with active lesions on nipple
- Hepatitis B or C and open wounds on nipple

Patient Education

- Expect an average of 8 to 12 feeds per day.
- Expect six to eight wet diapers and three or more stools by day 6 of life.
- Know that newborns may cluster some feeds together and go for longer periods afterward.
- Understand that newborns should not be on a set feeding schedule unless prescribed by the provider.
- Be aware that lactation requires an increase in your caloric intake (approximately 500 extra calories/day) and an increase in hydration.
- Continue to take prenatal vitamins during the entire time of breastfeeding.

BREASTFEEDING COMPLICATIONS

MASTITIS

- *Mastitis* is defined as localized, painful inflammation of the breast in conjunction with flu-like symptoms such as fever and malaise.
- Occurrence is approximately 10% of breastfeeding patients.

Signs and Symptoms

- Breasts that are painful, reddened, and hard
- Fever
- Malaise, fatigue, body aches, and/or headache

Treatment

- Improvement of breastfeeding technique
- Movement of milk by frequent emptying of breast through effective breastfeeding, mechanical pump, or hand expression
- Oral antibiotics or IV, if needed

Patient Education

- Wash hands prior to breastfeeding to decrease transmission of bacteria and prevent mastitis.

INABILITY TO LATCH

- If physical problems such as prematurity, reluctance to latch, tongue tie, or other issues affect inability to latch, the patient should be encouraged to express milk via hand expression or pump and use the expressed breast milk to feed the infant.

Lactation Support

- Assessment of readiness to feed in the premature infant
- Education of patients in proper pumping and milk storage technique
- **Until latch is established, AAP's milk preference for the newborn in the order of preference**: 1) mother's own milk, pumped or hand expressed; 2) donor milk from milk bank; 3) formula

FORMULA FEEDING

- The use of a commercially prepared, iron-fortified infant formula is another method of providing nutrition during the first year of life.

SAFE HANDLING

- Bottles of reconstituted powder formula may be refrigerated for 24 hours.
- Bottles of liquid concentrate or premixed formula are good for 48 hours in the refrigerator.
- Bottles, nipples, caps, and rings should be washed in warm soapy water followed by sterilization with commercial products or by placing them in boiling water for 5 minutes and drying.
- Bottles of reconstituted powder formula may be refrigerated for 24 hours.
- Caregivers should wash hands prior to mixing formula.
- Parents should not dilute formula as the nutritional needs of the infant could be compromised.
- Water to reconstitute powder formula should be boiled 1 to 2 minutes prior to mixing with formula.

BOTTLE FEEDING TECHNIQUE

- Hold infant during feeds. Never prop bottles.
- Hold infant in upright position for approximately 15 minutes after feeds.
- Never put a newborn to bed with a bottle due to risk of choking and neonatal collapse.
- Newborn's head should be slightly higher than the rest of the body so they may face caregiver for engagement. This upright positioning also prevents otitis media.

INHIBITING MILK PRODUCTION

Recommendations for the patient who is not breastfeeding are as follows:

- Application of cold packs to breasts
- Avoidance of nipple or breast stimulation (in severe discomfort, hand expression of a small amount of milk to relieve pressure)
- Application of cold cabbage leaves for pain and swelling
- Use of analgesics such as acetaminophen or ibuprofen for pain and swelling
- Wearing of a well-fitting bra

PARENT–INFANT BONDING

- Babies are very dependent on parents and caregivers.
- Brain, cognitive, and emotional development depends on attachment with a primary caregiver, usually a parent.
- Bonding is reciprocal and important for both caregiver and newborn.

ROOMING-IN

- The hospital policy of having infants room in with their parents allows for nonstop learning about the newborn.
- Rooming-in continues throughout the night.
- Rooming-in allows for up to 1 hour away for procedures or testing in the nursery setting.

SKIN-TO-SKIN CONTACT

- Skin-to-skin contact produces oxytocin in mothers, which further allows them to bond with their newborn as well as help milk production.
- Skin-to-skin contact can be done by parents as well as other caregivers and regulates newborn state, blood sugar, and VS.

SIGNS OF INADEQUATE BONDING

- An infant who cries inconsolably
- Lack of eye contact and smiling at baby
- Lack of response to infant needs such as hunger cues or need for diaper changes
- Parents not talking about their baby

Treatment

- Social service consultation should be ordered for concerns.
- These signs should be addressed with mental health professionals if seen while in hospital or outpatient.

PERINATAL LOSS AND GRIEF

- Parents experiencing a perinatal loss may react in different ways.
- The nurse must support the family in a range of possible emotions, from extreme sadness and crying to stoic behavior in which the family does not appear to grieve.

Nursing Interventions

- Refer to infant by their sex and name, if parents have given a name.
- Collect footprints, lock of hair (if appropriate), and photographs of newborn if the family desires.
- Encourage the family to spend time with the newborn and involve them in the collection of remembrance items if they desire.
- Suggest outpatient support groups and arrange follow-up calls by staff.
- Offer patient education on suppression of lactation.
- Refer to social services, chaplain, or religious leaders, as appropriate, to provide emotional support and assist with burial or cremation services if desired by the family.

RECOMMENDATIONS AFTER DISCHARGE

NEWBORN CARE AND SAFETY

- It is recommended to have quick a follow-up with a pediatric or family medicine provider within 2 to 3 days after discharge from the hospital.
- Newborns should not be on a set feeding schedule unless prescribed by the provider.

NEWBORN CARE AND SAFETY (continued)

- All infants should be fed on demand at least eight times per day, regardless of feeding method.
- Newborns may cluster some feeds together and go for longer periods afterward.
- Parents can expect six to eight wet diapers and three or more stools by day 6 of life.
- Newborns should be placed onto their back for sleep.
- Keep sleeping environment cool.
- Use a firm mattress with no soft bedding, bumpers, or soft toys.
- There should be no co-sleeping or bed sharing.
- Avoid secondhand smoke exposure.
- Avoid distractions, such as cell phone usage, while feeding and holding infant.
- Use pacifier after breastfeeding.
- Car seats should be less than 6 years old, should have never been in a crash, and should not have been recalled.
- Car seat should be appropriate for size and age.
- Parents should not use a car seat as a crib for sleeping; infants should sleep flat on their back in a crib.
- Do not use aftermarket "snugglers" or positioning products that do not come with the seat.
- The car seat should be placed in the back seat in the rear-facing position.
- **Circumcision care for male newborns include**: Apply petroleum jelly or dressing or gauze to area as directed to prevent diaper from sticking to wound, keep the area clean with warm water, and **report signs and symptoms of infection, such as significant increase in redness, bleeding, swelling, or pus**.

COMMON NEWBORN CONCERNS

Patient Education

- **Heat stroke**: Never leave a newborn alone inside your car. Infants do not have the ability to cool themselves and may die.
- **Shaken baby syndrome**: Forceful shaking can cause the brain to move back and forth inside the skull causing injury and should be avoided. Find calming ways to cope or relieve frustration, such as singing or gentle rocking. Normal play and gentle swinging are appropriate and will not cause injury. Most common cause of shaken baby syndrome is frustration from a caregiver because of infant crying. If you are frustrated and afraid you might shake your baby, it is always okay to put your infant down in a safe place and walk away to take a break.

Report any of the following signs and symptoms in a newborn:

- Blood in bowel movement
- Changes in color of skin
- Difficulty breathing
- Emesis with every feeding or brown- or green-colored emesis
- Fever or abnormal temperature
- Jaundice of skin or eyes
- Lethargy or not waking for feedings
- Odor, redness, or oozing from umbilical cord area or circumcision
- Unusual fussiness lasting longer than an hour

POSTPARTUM PATIENT CARE

- Analgesic creams
- Medicated pads and sprays
- Over-the-counter medications
- Prescription medications
- Deep breathing/relaxation techniques
- Donut cushions
- Hot packs for cramping
- Ice packs for perineal pain
- Massage
- Sitz baths

Patient Education

- Do not consume more than one alcoholic drink per day.
- Do not diet during the first few weeks of healing/postpartum period.
- Drink to thirst.
- Foods high in calcium, vitamin D, folic acid, and protein are recommended.
- Do not smoke. Infants can receive nicotine or marijuana in breastmilk or inhale chemicals.
- Smoking of any substance (tobacco, marijuana, etc.) can also increase the risk of SIDS.
- Exercise is not recommended until the first postpartum visit at 1–2 weeks.
- Begin with mild activity and work up to more vigorous exercise.
- Benefits of exercise include increased energy, reduced stress and improved mood, and reduced risk of postpartum depression.
- To lower risk of blood clots, walk around at least every 2 to 3 hours while awake and avoid crossing legs while sitting.
- Maintain vaginal rest for 6 weeks. Nothing should be inserted inside of the vagina during this time. This includes tampons, douches, fingers, and any type of vaginal sexual intercourse. All should be avoided during this time period.
- Pelvic floor/Kegel exercises are recommended.
- **Perineal care includes**: Relief of perineal pain with analgesics, ice packs, and sitz baths. Report foul-smelling discharge to provider. Rinse the perineum with a perineal irrigation bottle of warm water after each urination or bowel movement. Wash and wipe front to back. Pat dry.
- **Cesarean section aftercare includes**: Lift nothing heavier than the baby. Stair climbing and heavy lifting may strain the incision. Place a pillow to splint incision for coughing or sit-to-stand movements. Keep the incision clean and dry. Remove bandages per provider recommendation.

[ ] **COMPLICATIONS**

Most providers recommend that all postpartum patients follow up with their provider between 1- and 2-weeks postpartum and again at 6 weeks postpartum. This is to provide both medical and emotional support for the postpartum patient.

APPENDIX 5.1 MEDICATIONS FOR POSTPARTUM COMPLICATIONS

INDICATIONS	MECHANISM OF ACTION	CONTRAINDICATIONS, PRECAUTIONS, AND ADVERSE EFFECTS
Angiotensin-converting enzyme (ACE) inhibitors (lisinopril)		
• Cardiomyopathy, hypertensive disorders	• Relax blood vessels to lower blood pressure	• NSAIDs, such as ibuprofen (Advil, Motrin IB, others) and naproxen sodium (Aleve), decrease the effectiveness of ACE inhibitors. • Side effects include dry cough, increased potassium levels in the blood (hyperkalemia), fatigue, lightheadedness, headaches, and loss of taste. • Rarely, ACE inhibitors can cause some areas of the tissues to swell (angioedema). If swelling occurs in the throat, it can be life-threatening.
Beta-blockers (labetalol)		
• Cardiomyopathy, hypertensive disorders	• Relax blood vessels and slow heart rate	• Medication is contraindicated in patients with asthma, AV heart block, and hypotension. • Side effects include lightheadedness, low heart rate, and severe headaches.
Diuretics (furosemide)		
• Cardiomyopathy, hypertension, edema	• Each type of diuretic affects a different part of the kidneys • Help the kidneys release more sodium into the urine, decreasing the amount of fluid flowing through veins and arteries. This reduces blood pressure.	• Side effects include increased urination and sodium loss. • Medication can also affect blood potassium levels, causing either hyperkalemia or hypokalemia. • Other possible side effects of diuretics include dizziness, headaches, dehydration, and muscle cramps.
Antifibrinolytic (tranexamic acid)		
• PPH	• Blocks the breakdown of blood clots • Reduces bleeding and reduces the need for transfusion	• Side effects include nausea, vomiting, diarrhea, abdominal pain, and visual changes. • Rare occurrences of anaphylaxis have been seen.
Volume expanders (hydroxyethyl starch or hetastarch)		
• PPH	• Expands plasma volume	• Medication contraindicated in severe CHF and severe renal failure. • Side effects include wheezing, chills, flu-like symptoms, peripheral edema, headache, pruritus, and vomiting.
Prostaglandin E1 analogue (misoprostol)		
• PPH	• Stimulate contraction of the uterus to prevent or stop hemorrhage	• Medication contraindicated in patients who are allergic. • Adverse effects include diarrhea, stomach pain, nausea, gas, and vaginal bleeding.

(continued)

APPENDIX 5.1 MEDICATIONS FOR POSTPARTUM COMPLICATIONS (*continued*)

INDICATIONS	MECHANISM OF ACTION	CONTRAINDICATIONS, PRECAUTIONS, AND ADVERSE EFFECTS
Cyclic nonapeptide hormone (oxytocin)		
• PPH	• Stimulate contraction of the uterus to prevent or stop hemorrhage	• Medication contraindicated in patients who are allergic. • Side effects include nausea, vomiting, and more painful contractions.
Semisynthetic ergot alkaloid derivatives (methylergonovine maleate)		
• PPH	• Stimulate contraction of the uterus to prevent or stop hemorrhage	• Medication is contraindicated in patients with hypertension or in patients who are allergic. • Use caution when using with sepsis. • Adverse effects include hypertension, headache, abdominal pain, nausea, and vomiting.
Prostaglandin F2-alpha analogue (carboprost tromethamine)		
• PPH	• Stimulate contraction of the uterus to prevent or stop hemorrhage	• Medication is contraindicated in patients with asthma, acute pelvic inflammatory disease, or active cardiac, pulmonary, renal, or hepatic disease, or in patients who are allergic. • Adverse effects include fever, vomiting, severe diarrhea, nausea, flushing, headaches, and cough.
Antipsychotics (aripipazole)		
• Postpartum psychosis	• Rebalances dopamine and serotonin to improve thinking, mood, and behavior	• Grapefruit juice should not be consumed with this medication. • Medication contraindicated in patients who are allergic. • Side effects include headache, restlessness, dizziness, feeling unsteady, constipation, stomach pain, and increased salivation. • Report suicidal ideations or behaviors.

ACE, angiotensin-converting enzyme; AV, atrioventricular; CHF, congestive heart failure; NSAID, nonsteroidal anti-inflammatory drug; PPH, postpartum hemorrhage.

RESOURCES

American College of Obstetricians and Gynecologists. (2019a). Practice Bulletin 116: Management of intrapartum fetal heart rate tracings. *Obstetrics & Gynecology, 116,* 1232–1240.

American College of Obstetricians and Gynecologists. (2019b). Practice Bulletin 205: Vaginal birth after Cesarean delivery. *Obstetrics & Gynecology*.

Association of Women's Health, Obstetric and Neonatal Nurses. (2018a). *Fetal heart monitoring.* Position Statement.

Association of Women's Health, Obstetric and Neonatal Nurses. (2018b). *Continuous labor support for every woman.* Position Statement.

Association of Women's Health, Obstetric and Neonatal Nurses. (2018c). *Nursing care and management of the second stage of labor* (3rd ed.). Evidence based guideline.

Cunningham, F. G., Leveno K. J., Bloom, S. L., Dashe, J. S., Hoffman, B. L., Casey B. M., & Spong, C. Y. (2018). *William's obstetrics* (25th ed.). McGraw-Hill.

Decherney, A. L., Nathan L., Lauter, N., & Roman, A. S. (2019). *Current diagnosis & treatment: obstetrics & gynecology.* (12th ed.). McGraw-Hill.

Ladewig, P. A., London, M. L., & Davidson, M. R. (2017). *Contemporary maternal-newborn nursing care*. Pearson.

Landon, M., Galan, H., Jauniaux, E., Driscoll, D., Berghella, V., Grobman, W., Kilpatrick, S., & Cahill, A. (2021). *Gabbe's obstetrics: normal and problem pregnancies* (8th ed.). Elsevier.

Lawrence, R., & Lawrence, R. (2021). *Breastfeeding: a guide for the medical profession* (9th ed.). Elsevier.

Lyndon, A., & Ali, L. U. (2021). *Fetal heart monitoring principles and practices*, AWHONN, Kendall Hunt.

Miller, L., Miller, D., & Cypher, R. (2022). *Mosby's pocket guide to fetal monitoring: A multidisciplinary approach* (9th ed.). Mosby.

NCC. (2021). *Monograph: Fetal assessment and safe labor management*. Simpson, Kathleen, NCC.

Resnik, R., Lockwood, C., Moore, T., Copel, J., & Silver, R. (2019). *Creasy & Resnik's maternal-fetal medicine principles and practice*. Elsevier.

Simpson, K. R., & Creehan, P. A. (2021). *AWHONN's perinatal nursing* (5th ed.). Wolters Kluwer.

Tappero, E. P., & Honeyfield, M. E. (2019). *Physical assessment of the newborn*. Springer.

Troiano, N. H., Witcher, P., & Baird, S. (2019). *High-risk & critical care obstetrics*. Wolters Kluwer.

PROFESSIONAL PRACTICE

PROFESSIONAL ISSUES
Overview

- Issues of ethics, the law, patient safety, and quality improvement (QI) have important implications in obstetric nursing for the care of the patient and neonate.
- Decisions must be made ethically.
- High-risk scenarios have legal implications. Liability must be assessed.
- Patient safety must always be a priority.
- QI is an ongoing process to improve care.

ETHICS

Four principles are used to address ethical issues: Autonomy, beneficence, justice, and nonmaleficence

Autonomy

- *Autonomy* acknowledges an individual's right to hold views, make choices, and act based on their own personal values and beliefs.
- Informed consent requires that staff adequately inform a patient about their medical condition and available therapies.
- In order for the patient to make an informed decision, the provider needs to ensure that the patient understands all risks, benefits, and consequences.
- The patient then chooses whether they want the specific treatment(s).
- The provider must obtain informed consent via patient signature with a witness present.
- Respect for patient autonomy must consider both the pregnant patient and the neonate (or neonates), which may present conflicts between or among ethical principles. Example: A patient in labor initially refuses a Cesarean section. However, the fetal heart tracing reveals fetal bradycardia that does not improve with interventions. In this case, the provider states that the fetus will need to be delivered by an emergent Cesarean section, which places the ethical principle of patient autonomy in conflict with the ethical principle of nonmaleficence.

Other Ethical Principles

- *Beneficence* is doing good and providing care that benefits the patient. Example: The nurse caring for a patient in labor provides a massage to help with pain management. ▶

POP QUIZ 6.1

A nurse is caring for a patient who has developed a birth plan that includes delayed bathing of the neonate. The nurse tells the patient that they cannot follow the birth plan because the baby needs to be bathed right away. What ethical principle applies to this situation?

POP QUIZ 6.2

A nurse volunteers at a clinic for underserved patients. What ethical principle is the provider following?

Other Ethical Principles (*continued*)
- *Justice* is the principle of rendering to others what is due to them. Example: The medical staff can use a triage system to determine which patient receives care first.
- *Nonmaleficence* is an obligation to not cause harm or injury. Example: A nurse is working while impaired. It is the responsibility of any nurse working with the impaired nurse to report the behavior and risk.

LEGAL ISSUES

Liability
- *Liability:* An obligation enforceable by law.
- *Administrative liability*: Violation of regulation. Example: A nurse fails to renew their nursing license but continues to practice.
- *Civil liability:* Imposition of penalty in the form of payment or compensation to a patient who was harmed.
- *Criminal liability*: Imposition of imprisonment or fines for crimes committed by a provider. Examples of potential criminal liability include a nurse not providing the appropriate length of resuscitation for a deceased neonate or a nurse administering an erroneous form, type, or dosage of medication that results in a patient's death.
- *Statute of limitations*: The time frame after an incident in which the patient or patient's family may file a lawsuit. For example, for an injury to a child during childbirth, the statute of limitations can be as long as 18 years.

Documentation and Medical Records
- In all cases, documentation should be correct, complete, and timely.
- Insufficient or otherwise poor documentation practices can be used against a nurse in the event of a malpractice lawsuit.

Standards for Documentation
- Ensuring the correct chart is being used before entering any data
- Making sure all documentation reflects the full extent of a nurse's professional capabilities and the nursing process
- Charting patient care in real time whenever possible
- Charting preventive measures and/or necessary precautions used, such as bed rails
- Charting the time of medication administration, the route of administration, and the response of the patient
- Documenting as often as needed and with enough detail to tell the entire story
- Documenting any patient refusal to allow a treatment or take a medication and reporting the refusal to a manager and the patient's physician.
- Documenting information added after the fact as late entries, including the time and date
- Recording phone calls to physicians, including the exact time, message, and response
- Using complete descriptions

Examples of Unacceptable Documentation
- Charting care before it is administered (advance charting), which may be considered fraud
- Charting a symptom such as "c/o pain" without including information on how it was treated or managed
- Using unacceptable shorthand or abbreviations
- Writing imprecise descriptions, such as "bed soaked with urine" or "a small amount of blood" ▶

Examples of Unacceptable Documentation (continued)
- Altering a patient's record, which is a criminal offense
- **Charting what someone else said, heard, felt, or experienced**: This should not be done unless the information is absolutely critical. If needed, use quotation marks, and properly attribute the remarks to the speaker.

Informed Consent

- *Informed consent* is defined as the patient's choice to undergo a procedure or treatment. It is based on the patient's full understanding of what is to be done, its benefits, its risks, and any potential alternatives.
- Patients have the right to autonomy to accept or reject interventions.
- The components of informed consent include the patient's knowledgeable approval after they have been given complete, unbiased information about the proposed treatment or procedure, its purpose, who will perform it, its expected outcomes, its benefits, its potential risks, its alternatives, the benefits and risks associated with alternatives, and the fact that the patient has a right to refuse a proposed treatment or procedure.

Negligence

- *Negligence* consists of the concepts of duty, breach of duty, causation, and damages.
- *Duty* is to optimize patient outcomes and prevent patient injury.
- *Breach of duty* is the failure to meet the standard of care. This prevents fulfillment of the duty to prevent injury.
- *Causation* is the direct connection between the provider's failure to meet the standard of care and the patient's injury.
- *Damages* may result in monetary compensation for the patient or patient's family. A nurse may not be responsible for the payment of damages unless the weight of the evidence shows that the care provided by the nurse was not in accordance with the standards of practice. The failure to meet the standard of care must be a cause of the patient's injury, and the injury must be permanent and/or have resulted in death.

EVIDENCE-BASED PRACTICE AND QUALITY IMPROVEMENT

PERINATAL CORE MEASURES

- The *Perinatal Core Measures* are performance improvement goals set by The Joint Commission to achieve integrated, coordinated, and patient-centered care that provide best outcomes for uncomplicated pregnancies and births.
- In 2020, the Core Measures PC-03 and PC-04 were retired, leaving four current measures.

PC-01 Elective Delivery

- PC-01 measures the number of elective deliveries (for nonmedical reasons) prior to 39 completed weeks of gestation.
- **Methods for decreasing the number of elective deliveries (the goal is zero) include**: development of protocols to not allow induction prior to 39 weeks for nonmedical reasons, increasing patient education on risks of induction, such as increased risk of operative vaginal delivery, and increased rate of Cesarean section.

PC-02 Cesarean Birth

- PC-02 measures the percentage of Cesarean deliveries for nulliparous patients with a term, vertex, singleton pregnancy.
- **Methods for decreasing the primary Cesarean delivery rate include**: decreasing inductions in patients with low Bishop score, increasing nursing education and support to achieve optimum labor management, using labor dystocia checklists by providers to ensure adequate labor times.

PC-05 Exclusive Breastmilk Feeding

- PC-05 measures the percentage of term singleton newborns who receive only breast milk while in the hospital setting.
- **Methods for increasing the rate of breast milk feeding include**: giving no pacifiers until breastfeeding is well established, increasing staff education on benefits of breast milk feeding and breastfeeding techniques, offering prenatal education on breastfeeding during prenatal visits or with breastfeeding preparation classes, offering lactation consultant support (including follow-up after patient discharge), requiring a provider order for the use of formula, rooming-in for postpartum patients and newborns, and using donor milk from milk banks as supplementation for patients with decreased milk supply.

PC-06 Unexpected Complications in Term Newborns

- PC-06 measures the percentage of infants with unexpected newborn complications for term newborns with no preexisting conditions.
- **Methods for improvement of complications in term newborns may include**: education for best practices in forceps usage, improved resuscitation protocols, revision of infection workup protocols, and second-stage labor-management protocols.

QUALITY AND PERFORMANCE IMPROVEMENT

OVERVIEW

QI is a framework to help improve healthcare and care of the patient and include the following concepts.

- Establishing a culture of quality in your area
- Determining and prioritizing potential areas for improvement
- Collecting and analyzing data
- Communicating results
- Committing to ongoing evaluation
- **Spreading successes**: sharing lessons learned with others
- Determining what needs improvement by collecting and using benchmark data.

Methods to Ensure Quality Improvement

- Implement evidence-based guidelines.
- Improve outcomes.
- Use standardization within quality improvement (QI) to decrease deviation in results.
- Place a priority on encouraging communication, engagement, and participation by all stakeholders.
- Start with a small, multidisciplinary team that is vested.
- Start with small-scale changes.
- Use a standardized process, such as the PDSA cycle, to implement QI projects or measures.

 **POP QUIZ 6.3**

What is the process that can be used when implementing a QI project?

PDSA Cycle
- **Plan**: Determine what needs improving and how to make the improvement.
- **Do**: Implement the change that is needed.
- **Study**: Monitor the implementation, and determine what changes are needed.
- **Act**: Make appropriate changes, as needed.

POSTPARTUM HEMORRHAGE

Quantitative Blood Loss

- The American College of Obstetricians and Gynecologists recommends quantitative blood loss measurement in the immediate postpartum period to ensure appropriate treatment for postpartum hemorrhage.
- In studies, visual estimation of blood loss has been likely to overestimate actual blood loss when volumes are low and underestimate when volumes are high.
- Quantitative blood loss measurement has been shown to be more accurate than visual estimation.
- **Quantitative assessment of blood loss includes**: direct measurement of obstetric blood loss and cumulative recording of postdelivery blood loss.
- A multidisciplinary team is best suited for developing protocols for the assessment of blood loss.
- Protocols should include methods for both vaginal and Cesarean births

Hemorrhage Cart

- A previously established, a hemorrhage cart should be present on each delivery unit.
- The contents of the cart help provide immediate care for uterine atony or cervical laceration without members of the team leaving the room.

Recommended Hemorrhage Cart Items
- Hemorrhage medications
- Instruments such as vaginal retractors, weighted speculum, sponge forceps, long needle holders, large curettes
- IV start kit, angiocaths, IV fluids and tubing, and items for lab draws
- Sutures and vaginal packing
- Urinary catheter kit with urimeter
- Uterine suction device
- Uterine tamponade balloon

Massive Transfusion Protocol

- A massive transfusion protocol is a policy that facilitates early provision of blood products to critically injured or massively hemorrhaging patients.
- By setting up availability of easy-to-access blood products with one order or phone call, patients receive transfusions faster ,with fewer hospital resources.
- By initiating the protocol, there is an emergency release for blood products.

Risk Assessment

- Active bleeding
- Cesarean birth
- Forceps-assisted birth
- Hematocrit test (HCT) less than 30
- History of previous postpartum hemorrhage (PPH) ▶

Risk Assessment (*continued*)
- Known coagulopathy or prolonged activated partial thromboplastin time (aPTT)
- Large uterine fibroids
- More than four previous vaginal births
- Multiple gestation
- Placenta previa or low-lying placenta
- Platelet count less than 100,000
- Prior Cesarean section or uterine surgery
- Retained placenta
- Suspected chorioamnionitis or temperature greater than 100.4°F (38°C) with no known source
- Suspected placenta accreta, increta, or percreta
- Vacuum-assisted birth

INDUCTION PROTOCOLS
- Protocols for induction of labor increase the rates of nonoperative vaginal delivery and decrease the chance of complications, such as operative vaginal delivery.
- The Bishop score should be used to rate the readiness of the cervix for labor. A number ranging from 0 to 13 is given to rate the condition of the cervix. Cervical ripening should be considered with a Bishop score of less than 6.
- Once the cervix is ripened, it is reasonable to use either a lower dose oxytocin protocol or higher dose oxytocin protocol.

TIMELY MANAGEMENT OF SEVERE HYPERTENSION
- *Severe hypertension* is classified as a systolic blood pressure 160 mmHg or above or a diastolic blood pressure 110 mmHg or above.
- Hospitals should have protocols established to treat severe hypertension in patients quickly to prevent sequelae of stroke or seizure.
- The goal of the protocol is to have severe-range blood pressure treated within 1 hour of documented notification of the provider.

DECREASING RACIAL DISPARITY
- There are significant racial and ethnic disparities in maternal morbidity and mortality in the United States.
- Black patients are three to four times more likely to die a pregnancy-related death as compared to White patients.
- The implementation of safety bundles is an important step to improving care to all patients.
- Protocols, checklists, and simulation trainings encourage the same care to be given to all patients regardless of race or socioeconomic status.

POSTPARTUM WARNING SIGNS
- Bleeding that soaks through one pad per hour or blood clots the size of an egg or bigger
- Blurry vision
- Headache that is not relieved with over-the-counter medications ▶

POSTPARTUM WARNING SIGNS (*continued*)

- Incision that is not healing
- Obstructed breathing or shortness of breath
- Pain in chest
- Red, swollen leg that is painful or warm to the touch
- Seizures
- Temperature of 100.4°F or 38°C or over
- Thoughts of hurting oneself or someone else

Teaching all postpartum patients which signs or symptoms to immediately report to the provider may further decrease maternal morbidity and mortality for all patients and reduce health disparities.

RESEARCH TERMINOLOGY

Review of Literature

- A *literature review* is a comprehensive summary of previous research on a topic.
- The literature review surveys scholarly articles, books, and other sources relevant to a particular area of research.
- The goal is to present a baseline understanding of current knowledge on the topic and identify any gaps in the research.

Qualitative Versus Quantitative Design Study

- *Qualitative research methods include gathering and interpreting non-numerical data. Qualitative data includes*: cultural records, documents, focus groups, interviews, observation, and personal accounts and papers.
- *Quantitative studies* compile numerical data to test causal relationships among variables.
- **Quantitative data includes** database reports, experiments, questionnaires, and surveys.

Sampling

- *Sampling* occurs when researchers examine a portion of a larger group of potential participants and use the results to make statements that apply to this broader group or population.
- It is important to determine if the sample was chosen at random or nonrandomly.

Method of Study

The method of a study is simply the way in which the data is collected to answer a research question.

- The process of collection of data
- The type of research performed (basic versus applied, exploratory versus explanatory, or inductive versus deductive)
- How the data was analyzed
- Tools or materials used in research, such as surveys or questionnaires
- Rational for choosing the methods of the research

Types of Research

- *Basic research* develops knowledge or predictions.
- *Applied research* develops techniques or procedures.
- *Exploratory research* explores the main aspects of an under-researched problem.
- *Explanatory research* explains the causes and consequences of a well-defined problem. ▶

Types of Research (*continued*)
- *Inductive research* develops a theory.
- *Deductive research* tests an already proposed theory.

Methods of Data Collection
- *Primary data* are collected directly by the researcher through interviews or experiments.
- *Secondary data* are collected by someone other than the researcher, such as a government survey.
- *Qualitative data* focus on words and meanings.
- *Quantitative data* focus on numbers and statistics.
- *Descriptive data* do not control any variables.
- *Experimental data* control variables to determine a cause and effect.

Validity and Reliability
- *Validity* is the extent to which the results really measure what they are supposed to measure.
- A valid measurement is generally *reliable*: if a test produces accurate results, they should be reproducible.
- *Reliability* is the extent to which the results can be reproduced when the research is repeated under the same conditions.
- A reliable measurement is not always valid: the results might be reproducible, but they are not necessarily correct.

Mode, Median, and Mean
- Quantitative research methods often describe data using the terms *mode*, *median*, and *mean*.
- *Mode* is the value that occurs most frequently in a set.
- *Median* is the number that separates the higher half of a sample from the lower half. It is literally the middle number in a data set.
- *Mean* is the statistical average of the data set. The sum of all numbers divided by the number of values in the set.

Research Results and Discussion
- In the *Results* section of a study, the researchers will provide technical data collected.
- The *Discussion* section of a study evaluates and interprets the data.

Practice Change
- The purpose of research is to evaluate current medical practice and to research new patient care methods.
- New research should be used to create evidence-based practice in the obstetrical professions.
- However, practice change cannot occur if clinicians are unaware of the research that has been performed.
- Approaches to disseminate new research include presentation at professional meetings and publication in biomedical journals.

RESOURCES

Agency for Healthcare Research and Quality. (2020). *Section 4: ways to approach the quality improvement process*. https://www.ahrq.gov/cahps/quality-improvement/improvement-guide/4-approach-qi-process/index.html

Agency for Healthcare Research and Quality. (2021a). *Approach to improving patient safety: Communication*. https://psnet.ahrq.gov/perspective/approach-improving-patient-safety-communication

Agency for Healthcare Research and Quality. (2021b). *CUS Tool—Improving communication and teamwork in the surgical environment module*. https://www.ahrq.gov/hai/tools/ambulatory-surgery/sections/implementation/training-tools/cus-tool.html

American Academy of Family Physicians. (2002). *Basics of quality improvement*. https://www.aafp.org/family-physician/practice-and-career/managing-your-practice/quality-improvement-basics.html

American College of Obstetricians and Gynecologists. (2007; Reaffirmed 2016). Ethical decision making in obstetrics and gynecology. *Obstetrics & Gynecology, 110*(6), 1479–1487. https://doi.org/10.1097/01.aog.0000291573.09193.36

American College of Obstetricians and Gynecologists. (2009). Patient safety in obstetrics and gynecology. *Obstetrics & Gynecology, 114*(6), 1424–1427. https://doi.org/10.1097/aog.0b013e3181c6f90e

Austin, N., Goldhaber-Fiebert, S., Daniels, K., Arafeh, J., Grenon, V., Welle, D., & Lipman, S. (2017). Building comprehensive strategies for obstetric safety: Simulation drills and communication. *Obstetric Anesthesia Digest, 37*(2), 61–62. https://doi.org/10.1097/01.aoa.0000515726.29190.ef

Birth Injury Help Center. (2022). *How long do you have to file a birth injury malpractice lawsuit?* https://www.birthinjuryhelpcenter.org/birth-injury-statute-of-limitations.html

Brigham and Women Faulkner Hospital. (2022). *What is just culture? Changing the way we think about errors to improve patient safety and staff satisfaction*. https://www.brighamandwomensfaulkner.org/about-bwfh/news/what-is-just-culture-changing-the-way-we-think-about-errors-to-improve-patient-safety-and-staff-satisfaction

Centers for Medicare and Medicaid Services. (2021). *Quality measurement and quality improvement*. U.S. Department of Health and Human Services, Centers for Medicare and Medicaid Services. https://www.cms.gov/Medicare/Quality-Initiatives-Patient-Assessment-Instruments/MMS/Quality-Measure-and-Quality-Improvement-

Cheng, A., Grant, V., Dieckmann, P., Arora, S., Robinson, T., & Eppich, W. (2015). Faculty development for simulation programs: Five issues for the future of debriefing training. *Simulation in Healthcare: The Journal of the Society for Simulation in Healthcare, 10*(4), 217–222. https://journals.lww.com/simulationinhealthcare/pages/articleviewer.aspx?year=2015&issue=08000&article=00004&type=Fulltext

Harder, N. (2018). The value of simulation in health care: The obvious, the tangential, and the obscure. *Clinical Simulation in Nursing*. https://www.nursingsimulation.org/article/S1876-1399(17)30357-2/fulltext

Lippke, S., Derksen, C., Keller, F. M., Kötting, L., Schmiedhofer, M., & Welp, A. (2021). Effectiveness of communication interventions in obstetrics—A systematic review. *International Journal of Environmental Research and Public Health, 18*(5), 2616. https://doi.org/10.3390/ijerph18052616

OPLN Law. (2020). *Substandard quality of care: What you need to know*. https://lawnj.net/information/substandard-care

7 PRACTICE TEST QUESTIONS

1. A patient presents to the labor and delivery triage unit with reports of vaginal discharge. The provider collects a sample of the fluid and prepares a wet mount. The provider visualizes ferning under the microscope. Ferning is an indication of:
   A. Recent intercourse
   B. Rupture of membranes
   C. Sexually transmitted infection

2. A patient at 38 weeks' gestation with a history of two Cesarean deliveries presents to the labor and delivery unit reporting intense acute abdominal and shoulder pain. The fetal heart tracing shows a sudden onset of fetal bradycardia with recurrent variable decelerations and minimal variability. On physical examination, the nurse observes a change in the contour of the abdomen and palpates the fetus through the abdominal wall. The action the nurse should complete first is to:
   A. Administer morphine sulfate 1 mg as prescribed
   B. Continue to monitor the patient and document findings
   C. Notify the provider immediately

3. A patient with a prolonged second stage of labor is undergoing Cesarean delivery. The provider is having a difficult time delivering the fetus and asks the nurse to apply manual upward pressure to the fetal head, which does not succeed in helping to deliver the fetus. The next maneuver the nurse expects the provider to perform is:
   A. Leopold
   B. Patwardhan
   C. Zavanelli

4. A patient is admitted to the antepartum unit at 22 weeks' gestation with a cervix at 1.8 cm. The patient's last baby was born early at 30 weeks' gestation and is now 10 months old. The patient is not having uterine contractions, and a cervical examination reveals 1 cm dilated, 20% effaced. The nurse expects the provider to order:
   A. 24 hours of intravenous magnesium sulfate administration
   B. Intramuscular injection of betamethasone (Celestone) now and once again in 24 hours
   C. Weekly intramuscular injection of 17 α-hydroxyprogesterone caproate (Makena)

5. A pregnant patient presents to triage with bilateral lower extremity edema, fatigue, and dyspnea. The electrocardiogram is abnormal, and the provider orders an echocardiogram and a chest x-ray. After reviewing the results, the provider diagnoses the patient with peripartum cardiomyopathy (PPCM). The result that reflects the provider's diagnosis of this patient is:
   A. Cardiomegaly, pulmonary edema, and pleural effusion on x-ray
   B. Prolapse of the mitral valve on echocardiogram
   C. Right ventricular systolic dysfunction on echocardiogram

6. A laboring patient is augmented with oxytocin (Pitocin) after being 4 cm dilated for 6 hours. After 2 hours, the patient calls to the nurses' station to report a large amount of vaginal bleeding along with abdominal pain. The electronic fetal monitoring strip shows a fetal heart rate of 135 bpm with moderate variability and no decelerations, along with uterine tachysystole. The provider performs a digital cervical examination on the patient, which reveals a cervical dilation of 5 cm. The nurse now notes recurrent late decelerations on the electronic fetal monitoring strip. The nurse expects that the next order from the provider will be:
   A. Administration of terbutaline (Brethine)
   B. Discontinuation of oxytocin (Pitocin)
   C. Intravenous bolus of sodium chloride (normal saline)

7. A patient who is pregnant with monozygotic twins is in labor. Prenatal ultrasound has confirmed that there is one amnion, one chorion, and one placenta. On the electronic fetal monitor, the nurse sees a category 2 fetal tracing on twin B, with deep, recurrent, variable decelerations. This tracing would concern the nurse because:
   A. Twin B may be breech
   B. There could be meconium-stained fluid
   C. There is a risk for umbilical cord entanglement

8. The patient who meets the criteria for induction or augmentation of labor with oxytocin (Pitocin) is the patient who:
   A. Experienced spontaneous rupture of membranes with regular contractions and cervical dilation
   B. Had a previous vertical Cesarean incision
   C. Is group B *Streptococcus* positive (GBS+) with ruptured membranes

9. Follow-up phone calls after discharge, which allow the perinatal nurse to clarify information and answer additional questions, should be provided to the patient within how many weeks after birth?
   A. 3
   B. 4
   C. 6

10. A patient who previously expressed the desire to breastfeed has just delivered a healthy term newborn with an Apgar score of 8/9. The newborn is currently lying skin-to-skin on the patient's chest. The nurse provides the patient with breastfeeding education and explains that the newborn should be breastfed within how many hours of birth?
    A. 1
    B. 1.5
    C. 2

11. A patient presents to the labor and delivery unit for a scheduled induction of labor. The nurse places an external monitoring device on the patient's abdomen to assess fetal heart rate. This device is known as a:
    A. Doppler ultrasound transducer
    B. Fetal scalp electrode
    C. Tocodynamometer

12. A patient delivered a healthy newborn 30 minutes ago. Since delivery, the patient has had more than 1,200 mL of vaginal bleeding, blood pressure is 78/52 mmHg, and pulse is 125 bpm. There are no signs of retained placenta or lacerations. The provider has administered oxytocin (Pitocin), misoprostol (Cytotec), methylergonovine maleate (Methergine), and carboprost tromethamine (Hemabate). To resolve the patient's condition, the nurse expects the provider to order:
    A. Bakri balloon
    B. Blood pressure management
    C. Dilation and curettage

13. A patient presents to the labor and delivery triage unit at 32 weeks' gestation with reports of uterine contractions for the past 6 hours. The provider performs a sterile speculum examination. Upon visualization of the cervix, a clear fluid is seen escaping the cervical os. This indicates:
    A. Hemorrhage
    B. Leukorrhea of pregnancy
    C. Preterm rupture of membranes

14. A patient who is pregnant with monozygotic twins at 32 weeks' gestation has been admitted for inpatient monitoring. The nurse applies the electronic fetal monitor and cannot find a heartbeat for twin B. The provider confirms that there is no heartbeat for twin B. Twin A has a category 1 fetal heart rate tracing. The intervention the nurse would expect to perform is to:
    A. Prepare to transfer the patient for induction of labor
    B. Schedule the patient for a Cesarean section
    C. Continue to monitor the patient

15. A patient who is 48 hours postpartum reports a severe headache for the past 2 hours along with heartburn and intermittent right upper quadrant pain. The patient also reports having trouble eating and drinking due to extreme nausea. Blood pressure is 158/100 mmHg. This patient's likely diagnosis is:
    A. Dehydration
    B. Gallstones
    C. Preeclampsia

16. A patient is 34 weeks' pregnant and is admitted to the labor and delivery unit after arriving at the obstetrics emergency department with reports of decreased fetal movement. A nonstress test (NST) is ordered, and it is nonreactive. A biophysical profile (BPP) is ordered by the provider, which reveals an amniotic fluid index score of 0, a fetal breathing movement score of 0, a fetal movement score of 0, and a fetal tone score of 0. The nurse would expect the provider to order:
    A. Cesarean delivery
    B. Induction of labor
    C. Repeat BPP in 24 hours

17. A second-trimester transabdominal ultrasound reveals a low-lying placenta. Repeat screening is scheduled to be done at 32 weeks' gestation. The most likely finding on the third-trimester follow-up is:
    A. Low-lying status unchanged
    B. Progression to placenta previa
    C. Resolution of the condition

18. After the patient has been pushing for 2 hours, the nurse notes that the electronic fetal monitoring strip is showing signs of fetal distress. There are recurrent variable decelerations with each uterine contraction, and no fetal descent has been noted during the last hour of pushing with uterine contractions. The provider applies a vacuum to assist with vaginal delivery. After three pulls with the vacuum with no fetal descent, the nurse expects the provider to order:
    A. Cesarean delivery
    B. Forceps operative delivery
    C. Repeat attempt at vacuum operative delivery

19. A patient is admitted to the labor and delivery unit at 33 weeks' gestation for observation for uterine contractions. The patient is White, has had two previous preterm births, and has a history of smoking cigarettes. This patient is at high risk for preterm delivery because the strongest risk factor for preterm delivery is:
    A. Being White
    B. Having history of preterm birth
    C. Having history of smoking cigarettes

20. The nurse is caring for a patient at 34 weeks' gestation with a twin pregnancy who presented to the labor and delivery unit with a large amount of bright red vaginal bleeding and a headache. After obtaining the vital signs of blood pressure 168/92 mmHg, pulse 122 bpm, and respiration rate 20 breaths/min, the nurse suspects that the patient may require immediate care for:
    A. Abruptio placentae
    B. Anemia
    C. Preterm labor

21. The nurse is caring for a patient with monoamniotic twins at 33 weeks' gestation who is in the hospital for prolonged monitoring. The fetal heart tracing is category 2 and has not improved after resuscitative measures. The intervention the nurse would expect next is:
    A. Discharge to home
    B. Magnesium sulfate administration
    C. Prompt delivery

22. A patient is having a repeat Cesarean delivery at 39 weeks' gestation. The circulating nurse notes that the provider makes a low transverse uterine incision on the patient. This is also known as what kind of incision?
    A. Gridiron
    B. Pfannenstiel
    C. Rutherford

23. A patient is admitted to the labor and delivery unit at 35 weeks' gestation with reports of severe headache, nausea, painful uterine contractions, and a gush of bright red vaginal bleeding. Upon assessment, the patient's blood pressure is 172/100 mmHg. Which medication is contraindicated in this patient?
    A. Methylergonovine maleate (Methergine)
    B. Ampicillin (Omnipen)
    C. Magnesium sulfate

24. In planning delivery for a patient at 36 weeks' gestation diagnosed with placenta accreta spectrum, the nurse would anticipate:
    A. Administering intravenous iron to the patient prior to delivery
    B. Preparing for birth of a fetus with intrauterine growth restriction
    C. Preparing the patient for a vaginal delivery

25. A patient is in the second stage of labor and is experiencing a shoulder dystocia. The provider turns the patient to the Gaskin position. Next, the nurse expects the provider to perform the maneuver known as:
    A. McRoberts
    B. Ritgen
    C. Woods corkscrew

26. A patient at 34 weeks' gestation is admitted to the labor and delivery unit with reports of fever, chills, body aches, nausea, and painful uterine contractions. Upon assessment by the provider, the patient has costovertebral angle tenderness and a temperature of 101°F (38.3°C). The medication the nurse expects the provider to order to address the priority concern is:
    A. Acetaminophen (Tylenol)
    B. Ceftriaxone (Rocephin)
    C. Nifedipine (Procardia)

27. When reviewing the fetal monitoring strip for a patient in active labor who is receiving oxytocin (Pitocin), the nurse notices six contractions over 10 minutes and minimal fetal heart rate variability. The priority nursing intervention is to:
    A. Administer oxygen via nonrebreather mask at 8 to 10 L/min and elevate the patient's legs
    B. Continue with labor support because these are normal measurements during labor
    C. Turn off the oxytocin (Pitocin) immediately and place the patient in a side-lying position

28. While the nurse is providing contraception education as part of discharge teaching, the patient states that they do not want to take birth control while breastfeeding because they have read that breastfeeding alone will prevent pregnancy. The response by the nurse that addresses the appropriate contraception education is:
    A. "I am glad that you did your research. It sounds like you have determined the best method of contraception for you."
    B. "I understand that you will be breastfeeding, but this option may not be as reliable as other methods. Let's discuss the pros and cons of various methods."
    C. "That sounds like a great plan, but be sure to inform your provider about your choice of contraception at follow-up."

29. A postpartum patient has a history of deep vein thrombosis (DVT) due to a clotting disorder. As a measure to reduce the risk of reoccurrence, the nurse will encourage the patient to:
    A. Cross the legs when seated
    B. Rest in bed as much as possible
    C. Wear compression stockings

30. The nurse is caring for a postpartum patient who is 10 hours post Cesarean delivery. Responding to the call light, the nurse notes that the patient's pulse oximeter is alarming at 85%, and the bedside monitor shows that the patient is tachycardiac and hypotensive. The patient reports chest pain and is coughing incessantly. The nurse suspects the problem is:
    A. Cardiac arrest
    B. Pulmonary embolism
    C. Stroke

31. A patient is admitted to the labor and delivery unit for observation at 36 weeks' gestation after falling and landing on the abdomen. The nurse observes a sinusoidal pattern on the electronic fetal monitoring strip. The intervention the nurse expects the provider to order is:
    A. Cesarean delivery
    B. Induction of labor
    C. Maternal blood transfusion

32. A patient at 35 weeks' gestation is admitted to the labor and delivery unit for preterm rupture of membranes. The patient does not report any contractions at this time, and a cervical examination reveals that the patient is 2 cm dilated. There are no signs of infection. The medication the nurse expects the provider to order is:
    A. Betamethasone (Celestone)
    B. Magnesium sulfate
    C. Nifedipine (Procardia)

33. A patient with a twin pregnancy at 33 weeks' gestation has been admitted after experiencing contractions. Assessment reveals that the cervix is 3 cm dilated. The nurse would expect to administer:
    A. Corticosteroids
    B. Long-term tocolytics
    C. Magnesium sulfate

34. At 4 hours since delivery, the nurse notes central cyanosis in a newborn that worsens with crying and does not improve with supplemental oxygen. The nurse auscultates a heart murmur. With these assessment findings, the diagnosis that the nurse suspects is:
    A. Anemia
    B. Congenital heart disease
    C. Respiratory distress

35. The presentation associated with continuous labor support is:
    A. Decreased incidence of spontaneous vaginal birth
    B. Poor 5-minute Apgar score
    C. Shorter duration of labor

36. The nurse is caring for a patient who has anxiety and is 28 weeks' pregnant. The patient reports pain, but the nurse does not see any contractions on the monitor. The nurse believes that the pain is arising from the patient's anxiety. Four hours later, the patient calls out that the baby is coming. The nurse enters the patient's room to find that the fetus is crowning. The nurse calls for help, but help does not arrive before the baby is delivered. The nurse delivers the baby. The practice that puts the nurse at risk for liability is:
    A. Delivering the baby
    B. Waiting too long to call for help
    C. Watching the monitor for contractions

37. The provider orders intravenous ampicillin (Omnipen) every 4 hours for a patient admitted to the labor and delivery unit for preterm labor at 34 weeks' gestation. This medication reduces the risk of:
    A. Chlamydial ophthalmia
    B. Chorioamnionitis
    C. Neonatal group B *Streptococcus* infection

38. The nurse is caring for a patient who is laboring naturally. The patient is 5 cm dilated, at term gestation, with bag of water intact and no known complications. The nurse is performing intermittent auscultation for fetal heart rate (FHR) assessment every 30 minutes. The nurse places their hands gently on the patient's abdomen to assess fetal position for Doppler placement and to assess:
    A. Fetal activity
    B. Skin temperature
    C. Uterine activity

39. A patient had a Cesarean delivery 3 days ago and is about to be discharged. During discharge teaching, the patient reports experiencing swelling and redness around the uterine incision as well as purulent drainage from the incision. The patient also reports starting to feel feverish, with body chills and muscle aches. The nurse notes that the patient had a prolonged rupture of membranes before the Cesarean delivery. The patient's temperature is 101 °F (38.3 °C). The provider assesses the patient and decides not to discharge home today. The medication the nurse would then expect to administer is:
    A. Intramuscular ceftriaxone sodium (Rocephin) and oral doxycycline hyclate (Vibramycin)
    B. Intravenous amoxicillin (Amoxil)
    C. Intravenous clindamycin (Cleocin) and intravenous gentamicin (Gentak)

40. A patient is at 37 weeks' gestation with twins. The fetuses have discordant growth, so the patient has been admitted for observation with an electronic fetal monitor. Twin A has a category 1 fetal heart rate (FHR) tracing, while twin B has a category 3 FHR tracing. Based on these tracings, the nurse will prepare the patient for:
    A. Cesarean section
    B. Discharge home
    C. Induction of labor

41. The patient in labor has just received an epidural for pain relief. The nurse is at the bedside when the patient becomes anxious and complains of dyspnea. The nurse recognizes these as symptoms of:
    A. Epidural hematoma
    B. High spinal block
    C. Systemic local anesthetic toxicity

42. The potential outcome that may be seen when using hydrotherapy during labor is:
    A. Decreased blood pressure
    B. Increased risk of natural episiotomy
    C. Increased risk of perineal trauma

43. A patient in the second stage of labor needs a low forceps delivery. The patient does not have an epidural and is requesting pain medication before the procedure is attempted. The provider asks for a 20-gauge epidural needle and a local anesthetic. After locating the patient's ischial spine, the provider introduces the needle into the vagina and injects the local anesthetic. The nurse recognizes this procedure as a:
    A. Paracervical block
    B. Pudendal block
    C. Spinal block

44. A patient at 39 weeks' gestation is in the first stage of labor at 7 cm dilated. The patient reports painful uterine contractions and states being unable to tolerate the pain. The nurse expects the provider to offer:
    A. An epidural
    B. Intravenous fentanyl
    C. A pudendal block

45. A patient presents to the obstetrics emergency department at 35 weeks' gestation and reports decreased fetal movement for the past 2 days. A nonstress test is nonreactive. The patient is admitted to the antepartum unit, and an ordered biophysical profile (BPP) reveals a score of 6/8. The order the nurse expects next is:
    A. Cesarean section
    B. Discharge home
    C. Repeat BPP in 24 hours

46. Which statement made by the patient indicates an understanding of nitrous oxide and labor pain management?
    A. "I will wear the nitrous oxide mask throughout my labor."
    B. "My baby will be born sleepy."
    C. "My support person cannot hold the inhalation mask in place for me."

47. A patient at 19 weeks' gestation with their first pregnancy is diagnosed with asymptomatic placenta previa. The nurse will prepare to educate the patient regarding:
    A. Administration of antenatal corticosteroids
    B. Expectant management as an outpatient
    C. Hospitalization for tocolysis

48. The emergency department calls and requests a perinatal nurse to assist with the arrival of a pregnant trauma patient. The nurse anticipates that the:
    A. Patient resuscitation, if required, will focus on fetal outcome
    B. Patient should be placed on supplemental oxygen
    C. Patient should remain supine throughout the assessment if confined to a backboard

49. The hospital where a nurse works has analyzed data to compare its Cesarean section rates with those of other hospitals in the state. This process is called:
    A. Auditing
    B. Benchmarking
    C. Implementing

50. The characteristics of a pregnant patient who would be a candidate for intermittent auscultation (IA) for fetal surveillance during labor are:
    A. Preterm, having twins, with maternal gestational diabetes
    B. Term, with intact membranes, desiring hydrotherapy during labor
    C. Term, ruptured with clear fluid, on oxytocin (Pitocin)

51. A patient is admitted to the labor and delivery unit at 35 weeks' gestation with reports of intense itching of the hands and feet. The nurse expects the provider to order:
    A. Diphenhydramine (Benadryl)
    B. Hydrocortisone cream (Hydrocort)
    C. Ursodiol (Actigall)

52. A patient is admitted to the labor and delivery unit at 39 weeks' gestation for induction of labor for advanced maternal age. A contraction stress test (CST) with intravenous oxytocin (Pitocin) is ordered, and the patient has three contractions in a 10-minute period; no fetal heart rate decelerations are observed. The CST is considered to be:
    A. Incomplete
    B. Negative
    C. Reactive

53. The nurse is caring for a G3P0 patient at 41 weeks' gestation. The patient presents to the labor and delivery unit with painful contractions, stating that their water broke 12 hours ago. Meconium-stained amniotic fluid is noted on the underpad. The nurse places an electronic fetal monitor on the patient. A sinusoidal pattern is noted, but the nurse thinks it is likely a fetal sleep cycle. The nurse continues to admit the patient and finish charting. The nurse then becomes distracted by another patient who arrives in labor. When the nurse goes back to the first patient 3 hours later, the fetal heart pattern is still sinusoidal. The nurse calls the provider, who arrives on the unit and performs a STAT Cesarean delivery. The Apgar score is 1 at 1 minute and 3 at 5 minutes. The nurse's behavior can best be described as:
    A. Assault
    B. Battery
    C. Negligence

54. A 39-year-old patient is admitted to the labor and delivery unit at 37 weeks' gestation after a routine nonstress test for advanced maternal age is nonreactive. The provider has decided that it would be safest to deliver the patient at this time but wants to know if the fetus will tolerate an induction of labor. The test the nurse expects the provider to order is:
    A. Biophysical profile
    B. Continuous electronic fetal monitoring
    C. Contraction stress test

55. A pregnant patient with a history of seizures who is taking a new anticonvulsant medication arrives to the unit with preeclampsia. The interventions that the nurse will perform to prevent seizure activity in this patient are to:
    A. Avoid startling disruptions and encourage the patient to ambulate
    B. Encourage visitors and break up assessments throughout the day
    C. Place the patient in a private room and avoid startling disruptions

56. The nurse observes recurrent variable decelerations on the electronic fetal monitoring strip of a laboring patient. The provider performed an amniotomy 6 hours ago. The nurse can expect the provider to order:
    A. Intrauterine amnioinfusion
    B. Intravenous antibiotics
    C. Intravenous fluids

57. The most common cause of primary postpartum hemorrhage (PPH) is:
    A. Genital tract lacerations
    B. Retained products
    C. Uterine atony

58. A patient with a history of preterm delivery in the second trimester is seen in the obstetrics emergency department at 22 weeks' gestation with reports of vaginal spotting. The provider orders an ultrasound to assess the fetus and the cervical length. The ultrasound reveals a live intrauterine pregnancy with a fetal heart rate of 135 bpm, with no fetal anomalies observed. The patient is found to have a cervical length of 1.9 cm. The patient is admitted to the antepartum unit. The nurse expects the provider to order a:
    A. Biophysical profile
    B. Cerclage placement
    C. Contraction stress test

59. A patient is diagnosed with preeclampsia at 35 weeks' gestation and is admitted for an amniocentesis. Which ratio of lecithin to sphingomyelin indicates fetal lung maturity?
    A. 1:1
    B. 1.5:1
    C. 2:1

60. The delivery approach that the nurse would anticipate if a shoulder dystocia is suspected is a:
    A. Cesarean section
    B. Vaginal delivery with gentle downward traction of fetal head
    C. Vaginal delivery with restitution

61. After delivery of a newborn, the provider is applying gentle downward traction on the placenta when a cord avulsion occurs. After several attempts at a manual extraction, the provider is unsuccessful in removing all of the placenta. The patient begins to bleed profusely from the vagina. The next intervention the nurse expects the provider to order is:
    A. Bakri balloon placement
    B. Dilation and curettage procedure
    C. Uterotonic agents

62. A patient presents to the obstetrics emergency department at 33 weeks' gestation with reports of shortness of breath, swelling in lower extremities, and decreased fetal movement. Upon assessment, the patient has a blood pressure of 161/105 mmHg, 3+ pitting edema in the bilateral lower extremities, and a nonreactive nonstress test. The provider orders a biophysical profile that reveals an amniotic fluid index of 32 cm and an incidental finding of fetal ascites. The nurse expects the provider to admit the patient for:
    A. Blood pressure management
    B. Cesarean delivery
    C. Induction of labor

63. A patient with preeclampsia is 10 cm dilated and is instructed to push by the provider. While pushing, the patient begins to stare off into the distance. The nurse observes muscle stiffness and jerking movements in the patient's upper body. The patient's blood pressure measures 185/98 mmHg. The medications the nurse expects the provider to prescribe next are:
    A. Calcium gluconate (Gluconate) and lorazepam (Ativan)
    B. Hydralazine (Apresoline) and valproic acid (Depakote)
    C. Magnesium sulfate and labetalol (Trandate)

64. After knocking, the nurse enters a patient's room while the patient is breastfeeding and observes that the newborn's lips are flared outward, with an audible clicking sound during suckling, and that the newborn's nose and chin are touching the patient's breast. The observation that requires an adjustment is:
    A. Audible clicking sound during suckling
    B. Lips flared outward
    C. Nose and chin touching the patient's breast

65. An abnormal implantation of the placenta over the cervical os characterized by painless, bright red uterine bleeding is called:
    A. Placenta previa
    B. Placental abruption
    C. Vasa previa

66. A patient in labor has a fever of 101.2°F (38.4°C) and is reporting body aches and chills. The nurse observes fetal tachycardia on the electronic fetal monitoring strip. The patient came into the labor and delivery triage unit more than 18 hours ago with ruptured membranes and a closed cervix; the patient is now 7 cm dilated. The medications the nurse will expect the provider to order are:
    A. Intravenous acetaminophen (Ofirmev) and oxytocin (Pitocin)
    B. Intravenous ampicillin (Principen) and intravenous gentamicin (Genticyn)
    C. Intravenous sodium chloride (normal saline) and oral acetaminophen (Tylenol)

67. A patient is admitted to the labor and delivery unit at 33 weeks' gestation with reports of painless, bright red vaginal bleeding. Upon assessment, the electronic fetal monitoring strip shows a fetal heart rate with a baseline of 135 bpm, with moderate variability and no decelerations. No uterine contractions are noted. This patient most likely has:
    A. Placenta previa
    B. Placental abruption
    C. Placental insufficiency

68. The nurse will explain to the patient in labor why the patient's cervix must be assessed before administering an opioid analgesic by stating:
    A. "A cervical examination will allow me to determine what position the baby is in."
    B. "Opioid analgesics can increase your baby's risk of respiratory depression if they are given too close to birth."
    C. "The medication will provide less pain relief if it is given in early labor instead of more advanced labor."

69. A patient at 36 weeks' gestation and diagnosed with placenta previa arrives to the labor and delivery unit and reports that they have saturated two perineal pads in the last 30 minutes. The nurse notes a large amount of bright red blood on the patient's pants and underwear. The first action by the nurse is to:
    A. Call the provider
    B. Examine the patient's cervix
    C. Place the patient on a fetal heart rate monitor

70. Vacuum-assisted deliveries are associated with higher rates in the infant of:
    A. Cephalohematomas
    B. Cerebral palsy
    C. Sepsis

71. Operative vaginal deliveries increase the risk for:
    A. Cesarean delivery
    B. Perineal trauma
    C. Postpartum infection

72. A G6P5015 patient gave birth 30 minutes ago. The nurse is performing a routine fundal examination and notices a gush of bright red vaginal bleeding of approximately 300 mL. The patient's fundus is boggy and firms up only with vigorous massage. The most likely cause of this patient's bleeding is:
    A. Cervical laceration
    B. Retained placenta
    C. Uterine atony

73. The nurse provides a postpartum patient with discharge teaching regarding mastitis. The nurse instructs the patient to call the provider if the patient experiences tenderness, fever, chills, and the additional symptom of:
    A. Blurred vision
    B. Calf tenderness
    C. Hard, reddened mass

74. This month, the nurse has provided care during the birth of three sets of twins. The incidence of multifetal births has increased sharply over the past few decades due to:
    A. Increased prevalence of diabetes
    B. Lower maternal age at conception
    C. Use of assisted reproductive therapy

75. The nurse helps a postpartum patient breastfeed. The patient states, "I know I need more calories when I am breastfeeding, but I cannot remember what I learned in my prenatal class." The nurse knows that the number of additional calories the patient will likely need when breastfeeding is at least:
    A. 200
    B. 300
    C. 500

76. The most accurate information regarding the acid–base balance of the neonate at birth is obtained from the:
    A. Placenta lacunae
    B. Umbilical artery
    C. Umbilical vein

77. The provider orders magnesium sulfate for a patient admitted to the labor and delivery unit for preterm labor at 30 weeks' gestation. The patient has intact membranes, and the patient's blood pressure is 110/78 mm Hg. This medication will decrease the infant's risk for:
    A. Cerebral palsy
    B. High blood pressure
    C. Seizures

78. A patient at 39 weeks' gestation is currently in labor. Prenatal care has been normal during the pregnancy. The patient's sonogram on admission has shown an amniotic fluid index (AFI) of 4, and the nonstress test (NST) has been reactive. Variable decelerations are noted on the monitor as the patient progresses into active labor. These decelerations are most likely occurring due to:
    A. Cord compression
    B. Head compression
    C. Placental insufficiency

79. The nurse is caring for a patient who is pregnant with dizygotic twins. During delivery, the nurse would expect to see:
    A. One amnion, one chorion, and one placenta
    B. Two amnions, one chorion, and one placenta
    C. Two amnions, two chorions, and two placentas

80. The nurse sees a patient listed in the electronic medical records and notices that the name of the patient is the same as that of someone from the nurse's neighborhood. The nurse looks at the patient's chart to determine if the patient is their neighbor. The regulation this nurse violates is:
    A. Administrative Simplification Compliance Act (ASCA)
    B. Affordable Care Act (ACA)
    C. Health Insurance Portability and Accountability Act (HIPAA)

81. A positive Kleihauer–Betke test at 48 hours' postpartum indicates:
    A. Antibodies in the newborn's circulation
    B. Fetal blood in maternal circulation
    C. High levels of bilirubin in fetal circulation

82. A patient is admitted to the hospital at 37 weeks' gestation with severe headache, blurred vision, and blood pressure of 160/112 mmHg. Immediately after placing the patient on bed rest, the nurse will:
    A. Assess the patient's deep tendon reflexes
    B. Assess the patient's fundal height
    C. Obtain the patient's weight

83. The nurse observes late decelerations on a laboring patient's electronic fetal monitoring strip. This is most commonly caused by:
    A. Fetal head compression
    B. Umbilical cord compression
    C. Uteroplacental insufficiency

84. The nurse reviewing the electronic fetal monitoring (EFM) tracing for a patient presenting at 35 weeks' gestation with contractions knows that a category 1 tracing:
    A. Indicates fetal distress
    B. Strongly predicts fetal acid–base balance
    C. Suggests fetal metabolic acidemia

85. The nurse is caring for a patient who just had a vaginal birth after refusing an epidural. The provider is repairing a third-degree laceration, and the patient is crying and asking for pain relief. The ethical principle being violated is:
    A. Autonomy
    B. Justice
    C. Nonmaleficence

86. The labor support technique that is an example of cutaneous distraction is:
    A. Continuous labor support
    B. Music therapy
    C. Use of a birthing ball

87. A patient in labor reports a headache and nausea soon after receiving an epidural for pain management. The nurse observes recurrent late decelerations on the electronic fetal monitoring strip. The nurse begins to turn the patient to their left side and notices that the patient's blood pressure is 80/48 mmHg. The nurse expects the provider to immediately order:
    A. 10 L of oxygen via nonrebreather face mask
    B. Intravenous ephedrine (Corphedra)
    C. Intravenous ondansetron (Zofran)

88. The nurse is monitoring the fetal heart rate (FHR) of a patient at 28 weeks' gestation who is on the unit for 24-hour observation after a fall. Which FHR would cause the nurse concern?
    A. Baseline FHR of 165 bpm with increased accelerations and absent variability
    B. Moderate variability with frequent accelerations from baseline FHR of 155 bpm
    C. Variable decelerations from a baseline FHR of 160 bpm with minimal variability

89. The sign that the patient in labor is having difficulty coping with uterine contractions is:
    A. Inability to focus or concentrate
    B. Rhythmic, focused breathing
    C. Vocalizations such as moaning, chanting, or counting

90. A patient received an epidural for pain management and is now in the second stage of labor. The patient has been pushing for an hour without much fetal descent. After 2 additional hours of pushing, the fetal head is on the perineum, and the electronic fetal monitoring strip is showing fetal distress. To help expedite delivery, the nurse expects the provider to offer:
    A. Cesarean delivery
    B. Episiotomy
    C. Vacuum-assisted delivery

91. A patient who is at 30 weeks' gestation is admitted to the labor and delivery unit after several hours of painful uterine contractions. The electronic fetal monitoring strip shows moderate variability and several fetal heart rate accelerations that are 10 bpm over the fetal heart rate baseline, lasting for 10 seconds in a 20-minute period. The nurse interprets the nonstress test (NST) as:
    A. Reactive
    B. Nonreactive
    C. Inconclusive

92. What additional information can the nurse receive from use of electronic fetal monitoring (EFM) compared with intermittent auscultation (IA)?
    A. Heart rate
    B. Heart rate variability
    C. Heart rhythm

93. Accelerations of the fetal heart rate (FHR) at least 15 beats above baseline for a 15-second duration correlates highly with a fetus that has a(n):
    A. Abnormal acid–base balance
    B. Abnormal umbilical cord blood gas pH
    C. Normal acid–base balance

94. The parent of an infant born at 36 weeks' gestation asks the nurse why the obstetrician did not clamp and cut the umbilical cord immediately after the infant was delivered. The response by the nurse that indicates the benefits of delayed cord clamping for preterm infants is:
    A. "Delaying cord clamping for 30 to 60 seconds has several benefits for the preterm infant, including improved circulation and respiratory function and better blood flow to the brain."
    B. "Most obstetricians delay cord clamping on all newborns for 2 to 3 minutes to provide a higher blood volume to the infant and reduce the risk of the infant requiring blood transfusion."
    C. "Because your baby was born a little early, it is essential to delay the cord clamping so that the infant has additional time to begin breathing on their own."

95. A patient presents to the labor and delivery unit in active labor at 38 weeks and 2 days' gestation. The fetal monitoring strip shows the fetal heart rate decreasing during each patterned contraction and returning to baseline when the contraction stops. The action the nurse will take is to:
    A. Contact the provider
    B. Check the patient's cervix
    C. Continue to monitor

96. A patient at 41 weeks' gestation is admitted to the labor and delivery unit for a scheduled induction of labor. Upon assessment by the provider, the fetus is noted to be in a breech position. The nurse will expect the provider to perform:
    A. Cesarean delivery
    B. External cephalic version
    C. Forceps delivery

97. The nurse caring for a laboring patient is performing intermittent auscultation (IA) of the fetal heart rate (FHR). After palpating the abdomen to determine fetal position and uterine activity, the nurse listens to the FHR using a handheld Doppler. Once the FHR has been counted before, during, and after a contraction, the nurse will next assess:
    A. Blood pressure
    B. Radial pulse
    C. Respirations

98. A patient at 27 weeks' gestation presents to the emergency department reporting sudden onset of severe abdominal pain, cramping, decreased fetal movement, and vaginal bleeding. The patient reports recent cocaine use prior to symptom onset. On physical examination, the nurse observes midepigastric uterine tenderness, excessive vaginal bleeding on a perineal pad, and increasing fundal height inconsistent with dates. The anticipated diagnosis for this patient is:
    A. Placenta previa
    B. Placental abruption
    C. Uterine rupture

99. A patient is diagnosed with preeclampsia at 32 weeks' gestation and is admitted to the antepartum unit for a 24-hour urine protein test. The provider orders an umbilical artery Doppler velocimetry assessment, which reveals an abnormal umbilical arterial waveform. This assessment indicates:
    A. Fetal anemia
    B. Oligohydramnios
    C. Placental insufficiency

100. The provider performs a digital cervical examination on a patient who is at 39 weeks' gestation and in labor. The provider reports that they feel a fetal foot. The nurse would document the fetal position as:
    A. Breech
    B. Cephalic
    C. Transverse

101. A patient presents to the labor and delivery unit with grossly ruptured amniotic membranes. The patient lives 2 hours away from the hospital and reports spontaneous rupture of membranes 3 hours ago and decreased fetal movement since that time. Upon admission, a vaginal examination reveals a cord prolapse. The patient is taken to the operating room for an emergency Cesarean delivery. The 1- and 5-minute Apgar scores are 1 and 4, respectively. Cord gases are sent, and the infant is stabilized and transferred to the neonatal intensive care unit. The nurse predicts that the gases will reflect:
    A. Metabolic acidosis
    B. Respiratory acidosis
    C. Respiratory alkalosis

102. A patient at 37 weeks' gestation is admitted to the labor and delivery unit after being involved in a motor vehicle crash. The patient reports painful uterine contractions and vaginal bleeding. External electronic fetal monitoring is placed and reveals a fetal heart rate baseline of 60 bpm with a sinusoidal pattern. A sterile vaginal examination shows 1 cm, 20% effaced, −3 station. The nurse expects the provider to order:
    A. Cervical ripening
    B. Cesarean delivery
    C. Intrauterine fetal blood transfusion

103. A patient at 36 weeks' gestation with a history of aortic stenosis is inquiring about pain management options in labor. Based on the patient's history, the nurse would expect the provider to recommend:
A. Epidural
B. Nitrous oxide
C. Spinal block

104. A patient who delivered via Cesarean section at 38 weeks' gestation because of increasing blood pressure and a history of gestational hypertension was discharged home with their newborn 5 days ago. During a discharge follow-up phone call, the patient reports experiencing blurred vision as well as headaches that are not helped by medication. The patient states that it is probably due to the stress of being a new parent and inadequate sleep. What is the nurse's best response?
A. "I am sorry this time is stressful for you. Drink plenty of water and get a good night's rest to feel better tomorrow."
B. "You should call 911 or go to the nearest emergency department because you are experiencing a life-threatening emergency."
C. "You should call your healthcare provider immediately. You may be experiencing very high blood pressure that will need to be treated."

105. A patient with a history of previous preterm delivery is admitted to the labor and delivery unit at 33 weeks' gestation with reports of leaking fluid from the vagina and uterine contractions. The provider performs a sterile speculum examination and sees a stitch on the cervix that indicates:
A. B-Lynch suture
B. Cervical cerclage
C. Infection

106. The nurse provides a postpartum patient with discharge teaching about infections and fevers. The nurse instructs the patient to call their provider if they have an oral temperature greater than:
A. 37°C (98.6°F)
B. 37.5°C (99.5°F)
C. 38°C (100.4°F)

107. A patient is admitted to the labor and delivery unit at 29 weeks' gestation with reports of painful uterine contractions for the past 4 hours. The provider does a sterile speculum examination and visualizes the cervix to be approximately 4 cm dilated. The patient has a nonreactive nonstress test and has a biophysical profile (BPP) ordered. The BPP is 6/8 and reveals that the patient has oligohydramnios. The nurse will expect the provider to order:
A. Indomethacin (Indocin) and ampicillin (Omnipen)
B. Magnesium sulfate and 17α-hydroxyprogesterone caproate (Makena)
C. Nifedipine (Procardia) and betamethasone (Celestone)

108. The onset of copious milk production that occurs 48 to 72 hours after birth, when prolactin levels rise and progesterone levels fall, is known as:
A. Lactogenesis I
B. Lactogenesis II
C. Mammogenesis

109. A patient who was diagnosed with asthma in childhood delivered a full-term infant 2 hours ago and is now experiencing a postpartum hemorrhage. A medication to be avoided is:
    A. Carboprost tromethamine (Hemabate)
    B. Methylergonovine maleate (Methergine)
    C. Tranexamic acid (Lysteda)

110. The condition that is a known cause of polyhydramnios is:
    A. Duodenal atresia
    B. Intrauterine growth restriction
    C. Potter's syndrome

111. The nurse is caring for a patient in the operating room (OR) following delivery via Cesarean section for fetal intolerance of labor and failure to progress. After delivery of the neonate, the provider notes an abnormally adherent placenta. Uterotonics are being administered, and the patient is being warmed. The quantification of blood loss is 2,500 mL. The patient's pulse is 148 bpm, and the blood pressure has dropped to 96/32 mm Hg; the patient is unresponsive. The anesthesiologist has placed the patient on oxygen and is intubating and converting to general anesthesia. Another staff member has escorted the patient's partner with the newborn out of the OR suite and to the nursery. The nurse anticipates that the next step will be to:
    A. Initiate the massive transfusion protocol (MTP)
    B. Perform a Cesarean hysterectomy (C Hyst)
    C. Transfer the patient to the intensive care unit (ICU)

112. A patient is admitted to the labor and delivery unit at 32 weeks' gestation for observation for a shortened cervix after routine antenatal testing for a history of preterm delivery. A risk for preterm labor and delivery is indicated by a cervix of less than how many centimeters?
    A. 2.5
    B. 3.5
    C. 4.5

113. A patient with gestational diabetes at 41 weeks' gestation has been pushing for 2 hours, and the fetal head is delivered. With the next contraction, no progressive movement is observed. The intervention the nurse expects the provider to order next is a(n):
    A. Episiotomy
    B. McRoberts maneuver
    C. Zavanelli maneuver

114. A patient at 35 weeks' gestation reports abnormal swelling in the pelvic region accompanied by pain and difficulty breathing. An ultrasound reports the measurement of the amnionic fluid index (AFI) to be 50 cm. The fetus is observed to have an enlarged skull. The nurse should anticipate preparing the patient for an:
    A. Amnioinfusion
    B. Amnioreduction
    C. Amniotomy

115. A patient is admitted to the labor and delivery unit at 30 weeks' gestation for persistent headache, nausea, and severe-range blood pressure. The patient has a history of asthma and myasthenia gravis. Assessment by the provider reveals right upper quadrant tenderness and two beats of clonus bilaterally. The nurse expects the provider to order:
    A. Hydralazine (Apresoline)
    B. Labetalol (Trandate)
    C. Magnesium sulfate

116. A patient is admitted to the labor and delivery unit at 31 weeks' gestation with symptoms of preterm labor. The provider performs a digital cervical examination and finds the patient to be 4 cm dilated and 80% effaced with intact membranes. The patient is given betamethasone (Celestone) and nifedipine (Procardia). The medication the nurse expects the provider to order next is:
    A. Gentamicin (Gentak)
    B. Magnesium sulfate
    C. Misoprostol (Cytotec)

117. A potential maternal complication of multiple pregnancy is:
    A. Congenital anomalies
    B. Preeclampsia
    C. Preterm delivery

118. The nurse notes a prolonged deceleration of the fetal heart rate unrelated to uterine contractions and visualizes the umbilical cord at the cervical os. The priority intervention the nurse will perform is to:
    A. Prepare the patient for delivery
    B. Place a gloved hand in the vagina to elevate the fetal head
    C. Reposition the patient into a hands-and-knees position

119. A patient at 24 weeks' gestation who is diagnosed with oligohydramnios has experienced rupturing of the amniotic membrane. A fetal effect that may result is:
    A. Anemia
    B. Flexion contractures of the extremities
    C. Hypoxemia

120. During the third stage of labor after a vaginal delivery, the patient delivers an intact placenta followed by copious amounts of bright red blood. The nurse is unable to palpate the fundus abdominally and notices that the uterus is beginning to protrude out of the vagina. The patient is given a fluid bolus along with nitroglycerin (Nitrolingual). Next, the nurse expects the provider to perform a:
    A. Dilation and curettage
    B. Hysterectomy
    C. Manual reinsertion of the uterus

121. A term infant with thick, particulate, meconium-stained amniotic fluid was just delivered. The priority intervention that the nurse will provide during newborn resuscitation is:
    A. Continuous positive airway pressure
    B. Endotracheal suctioning
    C. Stimulation of the infant

122. A patient is admitted to the labor and delivery unit at 34 weeks' gestation with signs of preterm labor. Cervical examination reveals that the patient is 3 cm dilated and has intact membranes. The provider orders betamethasone (Celestone), 12 mg intramuscularly, to be given immediately and once again in 24 hours. This medication is given to help:
    A. Decrease inflammation
    B. Mature fetal lungs
    C. Prevent preterm birth

123. A healthy infant with an Apgar score of 9/9 was just born via normal, sterile vaginal delivery. After the cord is cut, the nurse immediately dries the infant and removes the wet towel. With these actions, the nurse is reducing heat loss due to the mechanism of:
    A. Conduction
    B. Evaporation
    C. Radiation

124. Advantages of using intermittent auscultation (IA) of the fetal heart rate, instead of electronic monitoring, during labor for fetal intrapartum surveillance include:
    A. Accurate tracing of fetal heart rate variability
    B. Greater patient mobility
    C. Need for less staffing in the unit

125. A patient with an antenatal diagnosis of placenta percreta is having a scheduled Cesarean delivery. After delivery of the newborn, the patient begins to bleed profusely. The provider initiates massive transfusion protocol and also orders uterotonic medications, which do not help to slow the uterine bleeding. The nurse expects the next procedure performed to be:
    A. B-Lynch suture
    B. Bakri balloon
    C. Hysterectomy

126. Compared with a neonate born through the vaginal canal, a neonate born via Cesarean section has a higher risk of developing:
    A. Cold stress
    B. Jaundice
    C. Respiratory distress

127. A patient has reached 33 weeks' gestation with a triplet pregnancy and reports feeling regular contractions every 6 to 8 minutes. The nurse would expect the provider to order:
    A. Corticosteroids
    B. Magnesium sulfate
    C. Tocolysis until full term

128. A patient in the first stage of labor has late fetal heart rate decelerations while supine. Lateral recumbent positioning affects the external electronic fetal monitoring device, and t cannot continuously trace the fetal heart rate. The provider evaluates the situation, and the nurse expects the patient to be offered a(n):
    A. Amnioinfusion
    B. Fetal scalp electrode
    C. Intrauterine pressure catheter

129. By 10 minutes of life, a term healthy newborn in extrauterine transition should reach a target oxygenation saturation (SpO_2) level of:
    A. 75% to 80%
    B. 80% to 85%
    C. 85% to 95%

130. A patient at 38 weeks' gestation with gestational diabetes is admitted upon accepting an offered induction of labor after an ultrasound that estimated fetal weight at 4,500 g. The fetus likely has:
    A. Hydrops fetalis
    B. Hyperglycemia
    C. Macrosomia

131. During a nonstress test (NST) for a patient at 39 weeks' gestation admitted to the labor and delivery unit for induction of labor, the fetal heart rate rises by 15 bpm above baseline for 15 seconds twice in a 20-minute period. This NST is considered to be:
    A. Nonreactive
    B. Positive
    C. Reactive

132. A patient is admitted to the labor and delivery unit at 41 weeks' gestation. The patient is 10 cm dilated, 100% effaced, and at +2 station. The fetal presenting part is the buttocks. The patient reports the urge to push and begins to bear down. The fetal body is delivered, and the head remains in the pelvis. With the next few contractions, the patient pushes, and there is no movement of the fetal head. If the body of the infant has been delivered for more than 2 minutes, the nurse would expect the provider to order a:
    A. Forceps-assisted delivery
    B. Symphysiotomy procedure
    C. Vacuum-assisted delivery

133. During the second stage of labor, a patient with gestational diabetes at 41 weeks' gestation with an estimated fetal weight of 4,000 g is having difficulty making adequate progress. The fetal head is visible at the introitus without moving the labia. The provider makes a midline incision down the patient's perineum to make room to apply a vacuum to the fetal head to assist with delivery. The nurse documents the midline incision as:
    A. Cerclage
    B. Episiotomy
    C. Ritgen maneuver

134. A patient has been in the second stage of labor for 4 hours. The fetal head is now near the perineum, but there is little to no fetal descent with each contraction. The provider decides to use forceps to help deliver the infant. This type of forceps delivery is:
    A. Low
    B. Midforceps
    C. Outlet

135. A patient with mild preeclampsia at 37 weeks' gestation is laboring and reports a headache. Upon assessment, the provider finds a blood pressure of 149/94 mmHg along with four beats of clonus bilaterally. The nurse expects the provider to prescribe:
    A. Ibuprofen (Motrin)
    B. Labetalol (Trandate)
    C. Magnesium sulfate

136. When using intermittent auscultation (IA) for fetal heart rate (FHR) monitoring, what would an auscultated FHR baseline of 110 to 160 bpm, a regular rhythm, and the presence of FHR increases with the absence of decreases in FHR from baseline be characteristics of?
    A. Category 1 auscultated FHR
    B. Category 2 auscultated FHR
    C. Category 3 auscultated FHR

137. A patient admitted to the labor and delivery unit for induction of labor at 41 weeks' gestation is given intravaginal misoprostol (Cytotec), and within 1 hour is having six to seven uterine contractions in a 10-minute period. The electronic fetal monitoring strip shows that the fetus is having late decelerations. Intrauterine resuscitation measures are started. The medication the nurse expects the provider to order is:
    A. Magnesium sulfate
    B. Nifedipine (Procardia)
    C. Terbutaline (Brethine)

138. The nurse caring for the patient in labor with suspected chorioamnionitis and noted fetal tachycardia on the electronic fetal monitor (EFM) tracing reports the findings to the oncoming shift. The oncoming nurse expects:
    A. That the provider will order an amnioinfusion
    B. To provide ongoing reassessment of the tracing
    C. Urgent Cesarean delivery due to fetal tachycardia

139. A patient in labor at 39 weeks' gestation is in the labor and delivery unit. The patient's lying blood pressure is 90/70 mmHg. The nurse's first action is to:
    A. Have the patient drink fluids
    B. Reposition the patient to their side
    C. Start an infusion of lactated Ringer's solution

140. A modified biophysical profile (BPP) is ordered for a patient at 37 weeks' gestation who is admitted after being involved in a motor vehicle crash. A modified BPP consists of:
    A. Fetal breathing and fetal movement
    B. Fetal kick counts and nonstress test
    C. Nonstress test and amniotic fluid index

141. The correlation of cigarette smoking with miscarriage can best be expressed as the following:
    A. Active maternal smoking has a damaging effect in the first trimester of pregnancy.
    B. Cigarette smoke contains toxins that directly affect the placental and fetal cells.
    C. Secondhand (passive) smoke exposure does not increase the risk of miscarriage.

142. The nurse is caring for a patient who is at 34 weeks' gestation with premature rupture of membranes (PROM). The patient asks why they are receiving antibiotics. The statement the nurse makes in response is:
    A. "Antibiotics with oxygen therapy help with the anticipated surfactant therapy of preterm newborns."
    B. "Antibiotics help reduce the infectious and gestational age–dependent neonatal complications."
    C. "Antibiotics are given to every laboring patient to reduce potential infection between the patient and fetus."

143. A patient presents to the labor and delivery unit at 32 weeks' gestation with reports of a large gush of fluid from the vagina and sudden onset of uterine contractions 45 minutes ago. The patient reports an urge to push. The provider performs a digital cervical examination and finds the patient to be 9 cm dilated, 100% effaced, and +1 station. The fetus is in a face presentation with mentum posterior. The nurse expects the obstetrician to order:
    A. Cesarean section
    B. Manual rotation to a vertex presentation
    C. Vacuum extraction

144. A Black G4P2205 patient is 36 hours post vaginal delivery of twins and reports shortness of breath when lying down to sleep. The patient also reports racing heart and swollen legs. Upon assessment, the provider auscultates fine crackles at the base of the patient's lungs posteriorly and anteriorly, and there is 3+ pitting edema in the bilateral lower extremities. The patient has a blood pressure of 98/50 mmHg. The provider orders an echocardiogram. The medications the nurse will expect to administer are:
    A. Furosemide (Lasix) and lisinopril (Prinivil)
    B. Magnesium sulfate and labetalol (Trandate)
    C. Nitroglycerin (Nitrostat) and warfarin (Coumadin)

145. The fetus of a patient who regularly uses marijuana is at increased risk of:
    A. Chromosomal irregularity
    B. Craniofacial abnormality
    C. Neonatal conjunctivitis

146. A patient is admitted to the antepartum unit at 30 weeks' gestation with a diagnosis of premature preterm rupture of membranes. The patient has a reactive nonstress test and has no signs of infection or labor at this time. Prophylactic latent antibiotics are started. The medication the nurse expects the provider to order next is:
    A. Intravaginal misoprostol (Cytotec)
    B. Intravenous magnesium sulfate
    C. Oral nifedipine (Procardia)

147. A patient is admitted to the antepartum unit for observation at 24 weeks' gestation with a monoamniotic-monochorionic twin pregnancy per recommendation by the provider. A routine nonstress test (NST) is reactive, and both of the fetuses are stable. The patient was diagnosed with type 1 diabetes at age 9 years, and this pregnancy was conceived through in vitro fertilization (IVF). The nurse expects the provider to order a(n):
    A. Biophysical profile
    B. Fetal echocardiogram
    C. Umbilical artery Doppler velocimetry assessment

148. During a nonstress test (NST) at 34 weeks' gestation, the electronic fetal monitor shows one acceleration of 15 bpm above the fetal heart rate baseline for 15 seconds once in a 20-minute period. The provider orders an additional 20 minutes of electronic fetal monitoring. During the additional 20 minutes, no further fetal heart rate accelerations are noted. The nurse can expect the provider to order:
    A. Additional electronic fetal monitoring
    B. A biophysical profile
    C. A fetal echocardiogram

149. A patient in labor reports feeling frequent uterine contractions. The nurse is unable to visualize contractions on the electronic fetal monitoring strip with an external tocodynamometer. The provider places a long catheter into the patient's uterus to better assess for contractions. This device is called a(n):
    A. Amniotic hook
    B. Bakri balloon
    C. Intrauterine pressure catheter

150. A patient diagnosed with placenta previa presents at 30 weeks' gestation with bright red vaginal bleeding. Fetal monitoring shows fetal tachycardia. The initial recommended action is to:
    A. Initiate tocolytics to prevent labor
    B. Place the patient on strict bedrest until closer to term
    C. Prepare for immediate Cesarean section delivery

151. A patient with no history of prenatal care arrives to the labor and delivery triage unit at approximately 35 weeks' gestation with reports of feeling a gush of fluid from the vagina. Upon assessment, the nurse observes grossly ruptured membranes with bright red vaginal bleeding. Electronic fetal monitoring reveals variable decelerations in the fetal heart rate. The patient is admitted for:
    A. Administration of corticosteroids
    B. Amnioinfusion
    C. Cesarean section

152. Accelerations of the fetal heart rate (FHR) are highly predictive of a normal fetal acid–base balance during the intrapartum period and can either arise spontaneously or be elicited by:
    A. Fetal scalp stimulation and vibroacoustic stimulation
    B. Palpation of the maternal abdomen
    C. Repositioning of the patient

153. A patient arrives to the labor and delivery unit for a scheduled induction of labor at 40 weeks' gestation. The patient reports no signs of labor, such as uterine contractions or rupture of membranes. The nurse can find fetal heart tones only near the fundus, and upon ultrasound assessment, the fetus is found to be in a breech position. The nurse expects the provider to initially order:
    A. Cesarean section
    B. External cephalic version
    C. Induction of labor

154. A patient is admitted to the labor and delivery unit at 33 weeks' gestation with reports of uterine contractions every 3 to 5 minutes. The provider performs a sterile speculum examination and visualizes a closed cervix with a small amount of thin, watery gray fluid in the vagina. A swab is collected for a wet mount. Upon inspection, the provider visualizes clue cells. The nurse expects the provider to order:
    A. Doxycycline (Vibramycin)
    B. Fluconazole (Diflucan)
    C. Metronidazole (Flagyl)

155. During continuous monitoring of a patient at 41 weeks' gestation, the nurse observes recurrent late decelerations. Late decelerations are directly related to:
    A. Fetal baroreceptor response
    B. Placental insufficiency
    C. Umbilical cord compression

156. A patient is admitted to the labor and delivery unit at 30 weeks' gestation with reports of painful uterine contractions for the past 4 hours. The provider performs a sterile speculum examination and visualizes a closed cervix. There is no bleeding or leaking of fluids noted. The laboratory test the nurse expects the provider to order is:
    A. Fetal fibronectin (FFN) swab
    B. Group B *Streptococcus* (GBS) swab
    C. Rupture of membranes (ROM) test

157. A patient at 35 weeks' gestation is admitted for observation after being involved in a motor vehicle crash. The patient does not report abdominal pain or uterine contractions, but the electronic fetal monitoring strip shows contractions once every 10 minutes. The patient reports bright red vaginal spotting after their last void. Laboratory workup shows a hemoglobin of 11 g/dL and a hematocrit of 34%, and the ABO/Rh is O negative. The nurse expects the provider to order:
    A. A blood transfusion
    B. Indomethacin (Indocin)
    C. Rho(D) immune globulin (RhoGAM)

158. A G6P4 patient with a history of postpartum depression delivered vaginally 26 hours ago and has just received the approval of the provider to discharge home. The patient calls the nurse and says that they are ready to leave. The patient has a referral for a social work consultation due to a high Edinburgh Postnatal Depression Scale score and a history of postpartum depression. The social worker informs the nurse that it will be another 2 to 3 hours before they able to visit the patient. The nurse will:
    A. Allow the patient to go home after they sign a form indicating that they are leaving against medical advice
    B. Cancel the consultation referral and give the patient the appropriate postpartum depression educational materials to take home
    C. Educate the patient on the importance of staying until the social worker can assess the patient and provide adequate resources to take home

159. A laboring patient at 38 weeks' gestation appears to have late decelerations on the electronic fetal monitoring strip, but it is unclear because uterine contractions are not being picked up well by the external tocodynamometer. The provider wants to place an intrauterine pressure catheter (IUPC) to obtain accurate visualization of the uterine contractions. Before the IUPC can be placed, the nurse will assist with a(n):
    A. Amniotomy
    B. Episiotomy
    C. Hysterotomy

160. A fetus with a reassuring electronic fetal monitoring (EFM) tracing is blue and limp upon delivery. The nurse stimulates the infant, and the infant takes a breath, turns pink, and screams. The nurse concludes that the infant experienced which acid–base imbalance?
    A. Metabolic acidemia
    B. Respiratory acidemia
    C. Respiratory alkalosis

161. After a successful external cephalic version in a patient who is at 39 weeks' gestation, the nurse's best expectation would be for the provider to order:
    A. Cesarean delivery
    B. Discharge home
    C. Induction of labor

162. Ultrasound examination reveals a trophoblastic attachment to the uterine wall without invasion into the myometrium. This type of placental disorder is known as:
    A. Placenta accreta
    B. Placenta increta
    C. Placenta percreta

163. A laboring patient with chronic hypertension suddenly begins projectile vomiting and reports a severe headache and blurry vision. The patient's blood pressure is 180/105 mmHg. Upon assessment, the patient has right upper quadrant tenderness. The nurse expects the provider to order:
    A. Blood urea nitrogen and complete metabolic profile
    B. Complete blood count with platelets and complete metabolic profile
    C. Protein-to-creatinine ratio and complete blood count with platelets

164. A patient is admitted to the antepartum unit at 22 weeks' gestation for hyperemesis gravidarum. An ultrasound reveals a fetal weight in the eighth percentile. The fetus has:
    A. Hydrops fetalis
    B. Intrauterine growth restriction
    C. Postmaturity syndrome

165. A patient presents to the labor and delivery triage unit at 38 weeks' gestation with reports of contractions for the past 4 hours. The provider begins to palpate the patient's abdomen, starting with a fundal grip. This type of assessment is known as:
    A. Fundal height assessment
    B. Leopold maneuver
    C. Manual palpation of uterine contraction

166. A patient in active labor arrives at the hospital. The patient has had limited prenatal care, has a positive toxicology screen, reports smoking cigarettes daily throughout the pregnancy, and reports a weight gain of 16 lb during the pregnancy. The nurse will expect the potential neonatal complication of:
    A. Fetal alcohol spectrum disorder
    B. Neonatal sepsis
    C. Small for gestational age

167. A patient with preeclampsia is admitted to the labor and delivery unit for an induction of labor at 37 weeks' gestation. Intravenous magnesium sulfate was started after several blood pressure measurements in the severe range. After 5 hours of induction, the nurse notices that the patient appears lethargic. Upon assessment, the nurse is unable to find deep tendon reflexes and notices that the patient has had a urine output of 20 mL since the last nursing round an hour ago. The patient's lungs are clear to auscultation bilaterally, and blood pressure is 138/98 mmHg. The nurse expects the provider to order:
    A. Discontinuation of magnesium sulfate
    B. Furosemide (Lasix) by intravenous push
    C. Intravenous hydralazine (Apresoline)

168. A patient at 38 weeks' gestation is laboring comfortably with an epidural. The most recent cervical examination an hour ago indicated that the patient is 7 cm dilated with the fetal head engaged in the pelvis. The nurse observes deep variable decelerations on the electronic fetal monitoring strip. When the nurse enters the patient's room for further evaluation, the patient is vomiting and reports sudden, sharp lower abdominal pain and a large amount of vaginal bleeding. A digital cervical examination reveals that the patient is still 7 cm dilated, but the fetal head is no longer engaged. The electronic fetal monitoring strip now shows a prolonged fetal heart rate deceleration of 80 bpm and uterine tachysystole. The nurse expects the provider to order a(n):
   A. Emergency Cesarean section
   B. Gaskin maneuver
   C. Vacuum extraction

169. A patient at 38 weeks' gestation with insulin-dependent gestational diabetes mellitus is being induced for labor. The potential complication that the nurse anticipates for the neonate is:
   A. Hyperglycemia
   B. Hypoglycemia
   C. Small for gestational age

170. A patient with no medical history and no previous pregnancies reports a headache for the past 2 days. The patient's vital signs are as follows: blood pressure 150/90 mmHg, pulse 80 bpm, respiration rate 16 breaths/min, temperature 98.7°F (37.1°C). The nurse asks the patient:
   A. "Have you experienced any epigastric pain?"
   B. "Have you experienced any numbness in your extremities?"
   C. "Have you experienced itchiness on your skin?"

171. The nurse is caring for a patient with a triplet pregnancy of 26 weeks' gestation. The patient reports fatigue, thirst, and frequent urination. Vital signs are blood pressure 110/64 mmHg, pulse 78 bpm, respiration rate 18 breaths/min, and temperature 98.6°F (37°C). When reviewing recent laboratory results, the nurse will expect to find:
   A. Elevated fasting glucose
   B. Elevated liver function tests
   C. Low hemoglobin

172. A patient is admitted to the labor and delivery unit at 35 weeks' gestation with reports of leaking fluid from the vagina for the past 24 hours. The patient also reports onset of fever and general malaise 3 hours ago that is unrelieved by over-the-counter acetaminophen. The patient reports mild uterine cramping since the onset of fever. Upon assessment by the provider, the patient has a temperature of 100.5°F (38°C), abdominal tenderness to light palpation, and grossly ruptured membranes with a foul odor. The cervical examination reveals that the patient is 6 cm dilated, 100% effaced. The nurse will expect the provider to order:
   A. Intravenous antibiotics
   B. Tocolytic agent
   C. Uterotonic agent

173. An evaluation of fetal growth reveals delayed growth in a pattern affecting the lower body and abdomen of the fetus, sparing head growth. The etiology indicated by the fetal growth pattern is:
    A. Aneuploidy
    B. Placental insufficiency
    C. Viral infection

174. Ultrasound screening at 20 weeks' gestation reveals that the edge of the placenta lies within 2 cm of the cervical os. This finding is indicative of:
    A. Low-lying placenta
    B. Partial placenta previa
    C. Placenta accreta

175. A patient presents to the labor and delivery unit in labor. The provider performs a cervical examination and reports that the patient is at 7 cm. This measurement refers to:
    A. Dilation
    B. Effacement
    C. Station

8 PRACTICE TEST ANSWERS

1. **B) Rupture of membranes**
   Ferning is a pattern visualized in amniotic fluid and can be seen on a wet mount with rupture of membranes. With recent intercourse, it is possible to visualize semen on a wet mount, but ferning would not be seen. With a sexually transmitted infection, moving trichomonas on a wet mount might be seen, but ferning would not be visualized.

2. **C) Notify the provider immediately**
   Uterine rupture refers to the actual separation of the uterine myometrium or previous uterine scar, with rupture of membranes and possible extrusion of the fetus or fetal parts into the peritoneal cavity. The patient with uterine rupture may complain of abdominal pain and tenderness and/or experience vomiting, syncope, vaginal bleeding, tachycardia, or pallor, as well as fetal distress. The priority for the nurse is to immediately notify the provider of this medical emergency to decrease risk of mortality to the patient and fetus. Subsequently, the nurse would administer morphine sulfate for pain, continue to closely monitor the patient, and document the findings.

3. **B) Patwardhan**
   The patient is experiencing an impacted fetal head during a second-stage Cesarean section, and the Patwardhan maneuver is a pull technique in which the provider uses a cupped hand to flex the fetal head while pushing upward toward the uterine incision as the nurse, or another assistant, uses upward pressure on the fetal head from the vagina. This technique has been shown to decrease both maternal and fetal complications. In the Leopold maneuver, the provider externally palpates the patient's abdomen to find the fetal position; this is not done during a Cesarean delivery. The Zavanelli maneuver is used during a shoulder dystocia to attempt to rotate the fetal head back into the pelvis; it would not be used in this situation.

4. **C) Weekly intramuscular injection of 17 α-hydroxyprogesterone caproate (Makena)**
   The patient would benefit from a weekly intramuscular injection of 17 α-hydroxyprogesterone caproate (Makena). This medication has been shown to decrease the risk of preterm birth in patients with a history of preterm delivery. The patient is at an increased risk for preterm delivery due to shortened cervical length, history of preterm birth, and short interval between the last pregnancy and this pregnancy. Intravenous magnesium sulfate is not indicated because this medication is used between the gestational ages of 24 and 34 weeks to reduce the risk of neonatal cerebral palsy in infants born prematurely, and this patient is at only 22 weeks' gestation. Intramuscular injection of betamethasone (Celestone), once now, and once again in 24 hours, is not indicated because this patient is at 22 weeks' gestation, and betamethasone (Celestone) to help mature fetal lungs is not indicated until the patient is at 24 weeks' gestation.

5. **A) Cardiomegaly, pulmonary edema, and pleural effusion on x-ray**
   A patient with peripartum cardiomyopathy (PPCM) may have cardiomegaly, pulmonary edema, and/or pleural effusions on x-ray. The patient may also exhibit left ventricular systolic dysfunction, with a dilated or normal left ventricle noted on echocardiogram. Mitral valve prolapse is a common complication in pregnancy, but it is not indicative of cardiomyopathy.

6. **B) Discontinuation of oxytocin (Pitocin)**
   The oxytocin (Pitocin) should be discontinued immediately for this patient because the electronic fetal monitoring shows signs of fetal distress, and the patient is showing signs of a placental abruption. An intravenous bolus of sodium chloride (normal saline) is part of intrauterine resuscitation and should be given, but the first intervention would be to discontinue the oxytocin (Pitocin) because that medication is the most likely cause of the uterine tachysystole, abdominal pain, and vaginal bleeding. Giving a tocolytic, such as terbutaline (Brethine), during a placental abruption is contraindicated because it can cause uterine atony and increase bleeding.

7. **C) There is a risk for umbilical cord entanglement**
   Monozygotic twins with one amnion and one chorion are at high risk for cord entanglement because the fetuses are in the same amniotic sac. Twin B may be breech, but that would not cause deep, recurrent, variable decelerations. There may be meconium-stained fluid because of fetal distress, but it would not be the cause of the deep, recurrent variables.

8. **C) Is group B *Streptococcus* positive (GBS+) with ruptured membranes**
   Patients who are GBS+ with ruptured membranes are excellent candidates for augmentation of labor. A patient with ruptured membranes who has not started labor will need augmentation with synthetic oxytocin (Pitocin) to reduce the risk of intra-amniotic infection. A patient who had a previous vertical incision of the uterus is not a candidate for a vaginal birth due to an increased risk of uterine rupture. The patient with regular contractions and cervical dilation is in labor and does not require labor augmentation.

9. **A) 3**
   Patients are typically in the hospital for 24 to 96 hours after birth, and teaching is provided in an inpatient setting. The American College of Obstetrics and Gynecology (ACOG) recommends that, after the inpatient teaching, all postpartum patients receive an opportunity to ask questions within the first 3 weeks after birth. Calling a patient 4 to 6 weeks after birth is later than ACOG recommends.

10. **A) 1**
    The nurse should explain to the patient that breastfeeding should be attempted within 1 hour of birth. Waiting until 1.5 to 2 hours after birth may result in unsuccessful breastfeeding goals for the mother-baby dyad.

11. **A) Doppler ultrasound transducer**
    The Doppler ultrasound transducer is an external device placed on the pregnant patient's abdomen that can transmit fetal heart tones. The fetal scalp electrode is an internal device placed on the fetal

scalp that can transmit fetal heart tones. The tocodynamometer is a device placed externally on the pregnant patient's abdomen that can detect uterine contractions.

12. A) Bakri balloon

The patient is experiencing a postpartum hemorrhage, which is defined as a loss of blood of 1,000 mL or more in a vaginal or Cesarean section delivery and is most commonly caused by uterine atony. Because medical management of the postpartum hemorrhage has not stopped the vaginal bleeding, a Bakri balloon is indicated to help compress the uterus. Blood pressure management is needed for this patient, but treating the cause and stopping the vaginal bleeding will help increase the blood pressure. A dilation and curettage (D&C) procedure is not indicated because there are no signs of retained placenta or membranes and the most likely cause of the patient's bleeding is uterine atony, which a D&C will not help.

13. C) Preterm rupture of membranes

Clear fluid escaping the cervical os is a sign of rupture of membranes. A patient at less than 37 weeks' gestation is considered preterm. Therefore, the provider is visualizing preterm rupture of membranes. A hemorrhage would consist of bleeding, not clear fluid, coming from the os or the vagina. Leukorrhea of pregnancy is a normal condition of a thin, white discharge from the vagina, not clear fluid escaping the cervical os.

14. C) Continue to monitor the patient

Prior to 34 weeks' gestation, if there are no other maternal or fetal indications for early delivery, the pregnancy should continue. Induction of labor or Cesarean section should be done at this time only if there are maternal or fetal indications for early delivery.

15. C) Preeclampsia

Preeclampsia is defined as a systolic blood pressure equal to or greater than 140 mmHg or a diastolic blood pressure equal to or greater than 90 mm Hg after 20 weeks' gestation, with either the presence of protein in the urine or systemic symptoms, such as severe headache, extreme nausea and vomiting, epigastric or right upper quadrant pain, visual changes, swelling in the extremities, or periorbital edema. Preeclampsia can occur up to 6 weeks postpartum. Dehydration may cause headache but would not explain high blood pressure or other symptoms the patient reports. Gallstones could be an underlying cause of right upper quadrant pain, but the overall assessment of the patient makes preeclampsia the most likely diagnosis.

16. A) Cesarean delivery

A Cesarean delivery is the most appropriate order because the biophysical profile (BPP) shows a score of 0/8. A score of 0 on a BPP indicates the need for immediate delivery because it suggests impending fetal asphyxia. A repeat BPP in 24 hours would be indicated for an equivocal score, such as 6/8, but waiting 24 hours to repeat the BPP could lead to an adverse outcome for the patient. Induction of labor would not be appropriate because the BPP score indicates impending fetal asphyxia. Not only would induction of labor potentially take too long to deliver the fetus, but the fetus may not tolerate an induction of labor since it is showing signs of distress and hypoxia.

17. **C) Resolution of the condition**
    Ninety percent or more of cases of low-lying placenta or placenta previa diagnosed in the second trimester are resolved by term. As pregnancy progresses, growth of the lower uterus brings about placental migration, with the edges of the placenta receding from the cervix, resolving the low-lying positioning and preventing progression to placenta previa.

18. **A) Cesarean delivery**
    The nurse can expect the provider to order a Cesarean delivery because an increased number of pulls during an attempted vacuum-assisted delivery can lead to increased risk for both maternal and fetal injury. It is generally recommended to stop attempts at an operative delivery after three pulls with no fetal descent, which is why a forceps operative delivery or a repeat attempt at a vacuum operative delivery would not be the best next steps.

19. **B) Having history of preterm birth**
    The strongest risk factor for preterm delivery is a history of a previous preterm birth. This patient has a history of two previous preterm births. Black patients, not White patients, are at increased risk for preterm labor and delivery. Smoking cigarettes does increase the risk for preterm delivery, but it is not as strong a risk factor as a previous preterm birth.

20. **A) Abruptio placentae**
    The patient is likely experiencing abruptio placentae due to preeclampsia. The bright red bleeding is a sign of abruptio placentae, while the patient's blood pressure and headache may indicate preeclampsia. The patient may experience anemia as a result of the bleeding, but a serious abruption may require immediate care. There is no indication of preterm labor.

21. **C) Prompt delivery**
    Monoamniotic twins are at an increased risk of umbilical cord entanglement. Delivery is usually recommended at 32 to 34 weeks' gestation. With an unresolved category 2 tracing at 33 weeks, an urgent Cesarean section will likely be performed. Discharge to home is not appropriate for a category 2 fetal heart tracing because there is no evidence of fetal well-being and there may be indication of cord entanglement. Magnesium sulfate is not recommended at 33 weeks' gestation because the benefits do not outweigh the risks.

22. **B) Pfannenstiel**
    This incision is referred to as a Pfannenstiel incision, and it is made in the majority of full-term Cesarean deliveries. It is an incision into the lower uterine segment about 2 cm above the pubis symphysis. A gridiron incision is a midline incision made down the abdomen, commonly used for open appendectomies or exploratory laparoscopies. A Rutherford incision is an oblique incision made on the lower right or left abdominal quadrant for surgeries such as renal transplantation or colon surgery.

23. **A) Methylergonovine maleate (Methergine)**
    Methylergonovine maleate (Methergine) is contraindicated in patients who are hypertensive because it can further exacerbate the condition and lead to a hypertensive crisis. Ampicillin (Omnipen) can be given to the patient and should be considered to prevent neonatal group B *Streptococcus* infection.

Magnesium sulfate should be considered to decrease the patient's risk of seizures associated with high blood pressure.

24. **A) Administering intravenous iron to the patient prior to delivery**
In patients diagnosed with placenta accreta spectrum, Cesarean delivery is typically scheduled. When iron deficiency is observed, supplemental iron is administered to increase preoperative hemoglobin. Placenta accreta spectrum is not a direct cause of intrauterine growth restriction. Vaginal delivery is contraindicated in patients with placenta accreta spectrum.

25. **C) Woods corkscrew**
The next expected procedure is the Woods corkscrew maneuver, in which the provider uses their hands to turn the fetal shoulder to an oblique position to allow more room for a vaginal delivery during a shoulder dystocia. It is often successful in resolving a shoulder dystocia. The McRoberts maneuver is performed when the patient is on their back. It involves lifting the legs to the patient's shoulder to help resolve a shoulder dystocia. This maneuver would not be the next logical step because the provider has already placed the patient in the Gaskin position, meaning that the patient is on their hands and knees. When performing the Ritgen maneuver, the provider uses upward pressure on the perineum to help control delivery of the fetal head. In this case, the fetal head is already delivered, so the Ritgen maneuver would not be performed.

26. **B) Ceftriaxone (Rocephin)**
The patient is exhibiting signs and symptoms of acute pyelonephritis. This upper urinary tract infection needs to be treated promptly because it can lead to maternal sepsis. The medication of choice is an intramuscular or intravenous cephalosporin, such as ceftriaxone (Rocephin). Acetaminophen (Tylenol) would help decrease maternal fever and chills, but it would be treating a symptom, not the infection that is causing the symptoms. Nifedipine (Procardia) can be considered because the patient is reporting painful uterine contractions, but treating the cause of the contractions, which is the infection, will be more beneficial.

27. **C) Turn off the oxytocin (Pitocin) immediately and place the patient in a side-lying position.**
The patient is experiencing tachysystole. The nurse's first step is to stop the patient from having more contractions by turning off the oxytocin (Pitocin) and placing the patient in a side-lying position. The nurse will then notify the provider and administer oxygen. Continuing with labor support is not recommended because the patient's contraction pattern is not normal

28. **B) "I understand that you will be breastfeeding, but this option may not be as reliable as other methods. Let's discuss the pros and cons of various methods."**
The nurse is correct to empathize with the patient regarding the worry about taking contraceptives while breastfeeding and to discuss the advantages, disadvantages, and misconceptions regarding the reliability of natural family planning in the postpartum stage. Consideration of the patient's needs and preferences is important, but simply congratulating the patient for their research and choice of contraception is not an appropriate response in this situation; the nurse should take the opportunity to clarify the patient's misconceptions and educate the patient on reliable methods. Telling the patient to let the provider know their contraception plans at their follow-up appointment is not appropriate because it does not include any opportunity to provide the patient with education regarding their options.

29. C) Wear compression stockings

Prevention of thrombus formation includes use of support stockings, early ambulation, leg exercises, correct posture, avoidance of crossed legs, avoidance of extreme leg flexion, decreased pressure on the back of the knees, and padding of pressure points. Patients with a history of deep vein thrombosis (DVT) will be encouraged to avoid crossing their legs and to ambulate frequently, and the patient will need low-molecular-weight heparin during their postpartum hospital stay.

30. B) Pulmonary embolism

A postoperative patient experiencing a pulmonary embolus may exhibit hypoxia, oxygen saturation of less than 90%, tachypnea, tachycardia, dyspnea, coughing, coughing up of blood, hypotension, confusion, fainting or collapse, or cardiac arrest. The patient is at very high risk for a blood clot because they are postcesarean delivery and have remained in bed for 10 hours postoperatively. The patient's symptoms are not representative of cardiac arrest or stroke.

31. A) Cesarean delivery

Cesarean delivery would be indicated because a sinusoidal pattern on an electronic fetal monitoring strip signifies fetal anemia and is considered a category 3 fetal heart rate according to the National Institute of Child Health and Human Development. It warrants immediate delivery. An induction of labor would not be the best choice for delivery because the length of time can vary for inductions of labor, and this situation requires imminent delivery. A maternal blood transfusion would not help with fetal anemia and is not indicated for this patient.

32. A) Betamethasone (Celestone)

The nurse can expect the provider to order betamethasone (Celestone) for this patient to help mature the fetal lungs. Studies show that fetuses up to 36 weeks and 6 days' gestation can benefit from corticosteroid treatment to increase fetal production of surfactant. Magnesium sulfate to reduce the risk of cerebral palsy in infants born prematurely is given between the gestational ages of 24 to 34 weeks, so it is not indicated for this patient. This patient does not have premature preterm rupture of membranes and is not in labor at this time, so nifedipine (Procardia) to try to slow labor down is not indicated.

33. A) Corticosteroids

Corticosteroids should be given, if possible, when there is a risk of delivery between 24 and 34 weeks' gestation. Long-term tocolytics are no longer indicated; only short-term tocolytics may be used to allow time for corticosteroids to be administered. Magnesium sulfate is indicated for neuroprotection in deliveries before 32 weeks' gestation.

34. B) Congenital heart disease

Central cyanosis and a heart murmur are the typical presenting signs of congenital heart disease. A newborn with anemia would usually have pale skin, not central cyanosis. With respiratory distress, crying would likely improve cyanosis by increasing oxygenation in the airway or lungs.

35. C) Shorter duration of labor
Continuous labor support by the nurse is associated with improved birth outcomes. Specifically, shorter labor, decreased use of analgesics, increased incidence of spontaneous vaginal birth, and higher 5-minute Apgar scores are associated with continuous labor support.

36. C) Watching the monitor for contractions
The action of a reasonable nurse would be to palpate the uterus for contractions. There are various reasons why contractions may not be seen on the monitor. The nurse should palpate for tightening of the uterus. The nurse acted reasonably when calling for help and delivering the baby. However, palpating the abdomen would likely have led the nurse to suspect preterm labor and to take appropriate action at that time.

37. C) Neonatal group B *Streptococcus* infection
Patients presenting in preterm labor at less than 37 weeks' gestation are at elevated risk for the potentially deadly neonatal group B *Streptococcus* infection (GBS). Ampicillin (Omnipen) every 4 hours may be ordered to prevent GBS. The drug is also used for the treatment of chorioamnionitis, but it is usually given every 8 hours in those cases. Erythromycin ointment applied to the neonate's eyes within 1 hour of birth is the preferred treatment to reduce the risk of chlamydial ophthalmia.

38. C) Uterine activity
Palpation of the uterus to assess contraction frequency, duration, strength, and resting tone is an essential part of monitoring the patient in labor. The fetal heart rate (FHR) must also be assessed before, during, and after a contraction to ensure that there are no signs of fetal intolerance of labor. The nurse may note fetal movement while palpating the abdomen, but that is not the purpose of the assessment. The skin temperature of the abdomen is not an essential part of the labor assessment.

39. C) Intravenous clindamycin (Cleocin) and intravenous gentamicin (Gentak)
The patient is presenting with signs of endometritis, the most common cause of postpartum infection. It is most commonly treated with intravenous clindamycin (Cleocin) and gentamicin (Gentak) while the patient is admitted. If not treated appropriately and swiftly, postpartum endometritis can lead to sepsis and adverse outcomes. Intravenous amoxicillin (Amoxil) is commonly used to treat group B *Streptococcus* infection while a patient is in labor, and intramuscular ceftriaxone sodium (Rocephin) and oral doxycycline hyclate (Vibramycin) are commonly used for outpatient treatment of pelvic inflammatory disease. These would not be first-line choices for postpartum endometritis.

40. A) Cesarean section
The twins are discordant, and a category 3 fetal heart rate (FHR) tracing is concerning because it is unclear how long it has been occurring. It is likely that the patient will undergo an emergent Cesarean section. The patient would not be discharged home with these risk factors. An induction of labor could occur if the FHR tracings were category 1 or possibly category 2, but induction agents cannot be given when a fetus has a category 3 FHR tracing.

41. B) High spinal block
High spinal block, near the level of the diaphragm, is associated with anxiety and dyspnea. Paralysis of the diaphragm leads quickly to respiratory arrest. Epidural hematoma is not associated with dyspnea but is suspected if lower extremity sensation does not return after discontinuation of regional anesthesia. Systemic local anesthetic toxicity is not associated with dyspnea. It typically presents with ringing in the ears, metallic taste, confusion, and, finally, seizure.

42. A) Decreased blood pressure
Hydrotherapy is an effective method of pain relief in labor because it promotes relaxation, decreases anxiety, and decreases pain. Additional benefits from hydrotherapy include decreased blood pressure, enhanced fetal rotation, and reduced risk of perineal trauma and episiotomy.

43. B) Pudendal block
This procedure is a pudendal block, used for pain control during the second stage of labor as an alternative to an epidural. This is a local block that numbs the nerves that innervate the S2 to S4 spinal cord, leading to pain relief in the sacral nerve area, including the perineum. It does not help with contraction pains but can provide pain relief during the second stage of labor or during a procedure such as a forceps delivery. A paracervical block is a local anesthetic block that helps numb the nerves that innervate the uterus and is commonly used during obstetrical procedures such as endometrial biopsy or hysteroscopy. A spinal block is a regional block done most commonly during a routine or nonemergent Cesarean delivery.

44. A) An epidural
The patient can safely be offered an epidural at this point. An epidural should be offered to decrease pain because the patient is in active labor, but delivery is not imminent. Intravenous fentanyl (Sublimaze) should not be offered at this time because the patient is a little too far along in labor for this medication. If delivery were to take place in the hour after receiving the medication, the infant could be born with respiratory distress. A pudendal block would not help with the contraction pain; it is best used when the patient has an imminent delivery and needs help with perineal pain, or if the patient will have an operative vaginal delivery and needs extra pain relief coverage.

45. C) Repeat BPP in 24 hours
A repeat biophysical profile (BPP) in 24 hours to reassess fetal well-being is indicated because the BPP score suggests that this fetus may be at risk for hypoxemia and requires further evaluation. A Cesarean delivery is not indicated with a score of 6/8, although it would be indicated with a score of 2/8 or less. The patient should not be discharged home because a BPP score of 6/8 indicates the need for further evaluation.

46. C) "My support person cannot hold the inhalation mask in place for me."
The patient should hold their own mask in place only when they feel it is needed. Nitrous oxide does not affect the fetus. Nitrous oxide is breathed in only during contractions, not continuously.

47. B) Expectant management as an outpatient

Patients diagnosed with placenta previa without bleeding, or asymptomatic placenta previa, may receive outpatient expectant management with serial antenatal ultrasounds to determine possible resolution of the previa. In the case of placenta previa with bleeding, antenatal steroids would be administered to the patient at less than 34 weeks' gestation, and the patient would be hospitalized and assessed for maternal and fetal well-being. The patient would receive tocolytic therapy for contractions.

48. B) Patient should be placed on supplemental oxygen

Protection of the patient's airway is of utmost importance. Oxygen supplementation via high-flow mask to maintain the patient's oxygen saturation at >95% is indicated even if no signs of respiratory distress are noted. Oxygen demands are increased during pregnancy, and with traumatic injuries, the demand increases further. When a pregnant patient is confined to a spinal backboard, they must be at a 15-degree left lateral tilt to prevent maternal hypotension from the compression of the vena cava by the gravid uterus and the subsequent decrease in uteroplacental perfusion. Initial evaluation and resuscitation of the patient take precedence over fetal evaluation. All efforts should focus on stabilization of the patient, which will also enhance fetal outcomes.

49. B) Benchmarking

Benchmarking occurs when outcomes are measured by an organization and then compared with the outcomes of similar organizations. Auditing is one way to measure the outcomes. Implementing is the process of making a change to improve an outcome.

50. B) Term, with intact membranes, desiring hydrotherapy during labor

Patients who are considered low risk for fetal hypoxia during labor are ideal candidates for intermittent auscultation (IA) for fetal heart rate monitoring during the intrapartum period. The term patient who desires hydrotherapy is the perfect candidate for IA because they are low risk and desire movement during labor, which the IA helps to facilitate. Contraindications to IA include the patient's being at higher risk for complications, such as when diabetes is present. Patients who are receiving high-risk medications, such as oxytocin (Pitocin), are not candidates for IA and must be continuously monitored via electronic fetal monitoring. Preterm and/or multiple-gestation patients are considered high risk and thus are not candidates for IA.

51. C) Ursodiol (Actigall)

The patient is reporting signs of intrahepatic cholestasis of pregnancy (ICP), which can manifest as intense itching, particularly on the hands and feet, and is caused by increased bile acids. Induction of labor is recommended for these patients starting at 36 weeks' gestation. Before then, ursodiol (Actigall) can reduce the patient's symptoms by decreasing circulating bile acids. Diphenhydramine (Benadryl) would not significantly reduce the itching because it would treat a symptom but not the root cause. Hydrocortisone cream (Hydrocort) can be used in patients with polymorphic eruption of pregnancy rash, which is usually found primarily on the abdomen, but it would not significantly decrease itching in patients with ICP.

52. B) Negative

The contraction stress test (CST) is considered negative because there are no fetal heart rate decelerations. It would be considered positive if fetal heart rate decelerations were observed. The CST is not incomplete because the criteria for the test indicate that the patient should have at least three contractions in a 10-minute period. CSTs are not described as reactive or nonreactive; *reactive* refers to a nonstress test that has two fetal heart rate accelerations of 15 bpm over the fetal heart rate baseline for at least 15 seconds.

53. C) Negligence

Negligence has occurred because a reasonable nurse in a similar situation would have called the provider immediately. It is unknown how long this fetal tracing was occurring, but it should have been addressed as soon as the nurse observed it. Battery is the intentional infliction of physical harm (e.g., striking a patient), and assault involves threatening to commit harm.

54. C) Contraction stress test

A contraction stress test is used to evaluate a fetus's response to labor. If the patient has at least three uterine contractions in a 10-minute period with no fetal heart rate decelerations, it is an indication that the fetus will tolerate labor well. If fetal heart rate decelerations are observed, then the provider may recommend a Cesarean delivery. A biophysical profile can assess fetal well-being but will not give insight into whether the fetus will tolerate the stress of labor. Continuous electronic fetal monitoring can assess fetal well-being, especially if the fetus demonstrates accelerations and has moderate variability in the heart rate, but if there are no uterine contractions, it is not an accurate predictor of how the fetus will tolerate labor.

55. C) Place the patient in a private room and avoid startling disruptions

Preventive seizure interventions minimize the amount of stimulation in the environment that could trigger seizure activity. These include placing the patient in a quiet, private room; avoiding startling disruptions; and minimizing light and noise. Rather than encouraging visits from family and friends, the nurse will restrict the number of visitors the patient receives. To further minimize disruptions, the nurse will also group assessments and patient care together rather than break them up throughout the day.

56. A) Intrauterine amnioinfusion

An intrauterine amnioinfusion can help decrease variable decelerations in the fetal heart rate by adding fluid around the fetus to help cushion the fetus and decrease umbilical cord compression. Intravenous antibiotics would not be needed because the patient is not showing any signs of infection. Intravenous fluids would help with late fetal heart rate decelerations to increase maternal blood volume, thereby increasing delivery of oxygen to the fetus, but they would not help to decrease variable fetal heart rate decelerations.

57. C) Uterine atony

The etiology of primary postpartum hemorrhage (PPH) can be categorized as primary (early: within 24 hours of delivery) or secondary (late: more than 24 hours up to 12 weeks after delivery). Uterine atony is the most common cause of primary PPH, and it is responsible for up to 80% of postpartum hemorrhage cases. Genital tract lacerations are a significant contributor to PPH, but they cause fewer cases than uterine atony causes. Retained products of conception (placenta or amniotic membranes) contribute to only 0.5% to 1% of cases.

58. B) Cerclage placement

The nurse can expect the provider to order a cerclage placement. This patient has a history of preterm delivery and is showing signs of a shortened cervix, which is defined as a cervix of less than 2.5 cm. The fetus has no apparent anomalies and has no signs of fetal distress, so a cerclage to help maintain the integrity of the cervix and to prolong the pregnancy is indicated. A biophysical profile is not the best course of action for this patient because antenatal testing is not indicated until at least 24 weeks' gestation to assess for fetal well-being. A contraction stress test is not indicated because the patient's current situation does not suggest a need for induction of labor.

59. C) 2:1

An amniocentesis to assess for fetal well-being and lung maturity can be performed when patient complications may warrant premature delivery of the fetus. A ratio of lecithin to sphingomyelin, which are phospholipids in fetal lungs that produce surfactant, indicates fetal lung maturity at a ratio of 2:1. A ratio of 2:1 or higher signifies fetal lung maturity. Before lung maturity, a ratio of less than 2:1, such as 1:1 or 1.5:1, may be present. A fetus born with this ratio is at increased risk for respiratory distress syndrome.

60. B) Vaginal delivery with gentle downward traction of fetal head

If a shoulder dystocia is suspected, it is appropriate to proceed directly with gentle downward traction of the fetal head before restitution occurs. When the fetal head crowns and delivery is imminent, gentle pressure should be used to maintain the fetal head's flexion and control delivery. Once the fetal head is delivered, external rotation (restitution) is allowed. A Cesarean section is indicated for cephalopelvic disproportion, placental abruption, placenta previa, repeat Cesarean delivery, Cesarean delivery on patient request, specific patient cardiac disease, nonreassuring fetal status, breech or transverse lie, and/or maternal herpes.

61. B) Dilation and curettage procedure

The patient has retained placental parts and needs to have them removed to reduce the bleeding, so a dilation and curettage (D&C) procedure would be the most appropriate intervention for this patient. A Bakri balloon placement would not stop the bleeding because it is due to the retained placenta. Uterotonic agents can be administered, but the goal is to stop the bleeding at its source—in this case, retained placenta—so uterotonic agents would not be the most appropriate treatment.

62. B) Cesarean delivery

Cesarean delivery is ordered because this patient is showing signs of Ballantyne syndrome, or mirror syndrome, which is a condition in which the fetus has developed hydrops fetalis. Hydrops fetalis causes edema in at least two different fetal compartments, including polyhydramnios, and the pregnant patient develops similar characteristics, such as edema or preeclampsia. Blood pressure management would be initiated as well, but it is not the primary course of action for this patient because waiting for blood pressure to be controlled before proceeding with a Cesarean section can lead to an increase in severity of symptoms for both the patient and the fetus. Induction of labor is not the best choice because Ballantyne syndrome is a life-threatening condition that requires immediate delivery.

63. C) Magnesium sulfate and labetalol (Trandate)

Magnesium sulfate and labetalol (Trandate) should be given to this patient immediately because they are exhibiting symptoms of a tonic-clonic seizure, which indicates that preeclampsia has progressed to eclampsia. These medications will help stop the seizure and decrease the risk of seizure recurrence as well as lower the severe-range blood pressure. Calcium gluconate (Gluconate) is not indicated because the patient is not showing symptoms of magnesium sulfate toxicity, and while lorazepam (Ativan) can be considered, it is not first-line treatment for eclamptic seizure management. Hydralazine (Apresoline) can be given for blood pressure management, but valproic acid (Depakote) is an anticonvulsant that is contraindicated in pregnancy.

64. A) Audible clicking sound during suckling
To verify proper latch-on and milk transfer, the following should be observed in the newborn: lips flared outward, absent clicking sounds, absent dimpled cheeks, moving muscles above and in front of the ears, chin and nose touching the patient's breast, most of the areola covered by the newborn's mouth, and wide angle of the newborn's mouth. Audible clicking sounds are a sign of an incorrect latch and require an adjustment.

65. A) Placenta previa
Abnormal placental implantation presenting with painless, bright red uterine bleeding that occurs during the second or third trimester characterizes placenta previa. With a placental abruption, the patient presents with sharp, stabbing, midepigastric pain that may or may not be accompanied by dark red vaginal bleeding. With vasa previa, the patient presents with vaginal bleeding that occurs during labor and that does not begin until after the rupture of amniotic membranes.

66. B) Intravenous ampicillin (Principen) and intravenous gentamicin (Genticyn)
This patient is exhibiting several signs of chorioamnionitis, an infection in the amniotic fluid, including fever, chills, body aches, and fetal tachycardia. Intravenous ampicillin (Principen) and intravenous gentamicin (Genticyn) are the first-line medications of choice to treat chorioamnionitis. Intravenous acetaminophen will treat symptoms of chorioamnionitis, but not the cause, which is usually a bacterial infection. Oxytocin (Pitocin) is not indicated because the patient is making adequate cervical change in labor. Intravenous sodium chloride (normal saline) and oral acetaminophen (Tylenol) may help decrease symptoms of chorioamnionitis, such as maternal fever and fetal tachycardia, but they will not treat the infection.

67. A) Placenta previa
This patient is exhibiting signs of placenta previa, in which the placenta covers the cervical os. Placenta previa can manifest as painless, bright red vaginal bleeding. Uterine contractions may not be present. In a placental abruption, the patient will have painful uterine contractions with bright red vaginal bleeding. Placental insufficiency would not manifest with bright red vaginal bleeding and would usually reflect fetal distress on the electronic fetal monitoring strip, which this patient does not exhibit.

68. B) "Opioid analgesics can increase your baby's risk of respiratory depression if they are given too close to birth."
The timing of the administration of opioid analgesics relative to the birth is associated with the level of risk of adverse effects like respiratory depression. Giving opioid medication within 2 to 3 hours of birth poses the greatest risk to the infant; therefore, the nurse should withhold the medication if the patient is more than 7 cm dilated. The baby's position is not related to the safety or efficacy of opioid analgesic use in labor; likewise, the labor stage does not affect the medication's effectiveness.

69. C) Place the patient on a fetal heart rate monitor

Painless, bright red bleeding can occur at any stage of pregnancy in placenta previa and is not necessarily a cause for alarm. The nurse's first action will be to check the stability of the fetus by analyzing the fetal heart rate. Calling the provider is important but is not the first nursing priority. Placenta previa is a contraindication for a cervical examination due to the risk of increased vaginal bleeding.

70. A) Cephalohematomas

Vacuum-assisted deliveries are associated with higher rates of cephalohematomas in the infant when compared with both forceps-assisted deliveries and spontaneous vaginal deliveries. The increased pressure on the scalp from the vacuum can cause blood vessels to break and cause a harmless collection of blood underneath the scalp. Vacuum-assisted deliveries do not cause a higher rate of cerebral palsy in the infant. Cerebral palsy is more prevalent in preterm infants or in infants who had a shoulder dystocia during delivery. Vacuum-assisted deliveries do not cause a higher rate of sepsis in the infant, although if there is a cephalohematoma present, it can cause an increased risk of hyperbilirubinemia.

71. B) Perineal trauma

Operative vaginal deliveries increase the risk of perineal trauma, including third- and fourth-degree lacerations along with anal sphincter injury. Operative vaginal deliveries decrease the Cesarean delivery rates in patients. Postpartum infections in operative vaginal deliveries are decreased when compared with Cesarean deliveries, which is the true alternative to a vaginal operative delivery.

72. C) Uterine atony

Uterine atony is one of the leading causes of postpartum hemorrhage. A patient is at higher risk for uterine atony with more than four deliveries. Uterine atony presents as a boggy fundus instead of a firm fundus after delivery. A cervical laceration could be the cause of the patient's bleeding, but the boggy fundus suggests that uterine atony is more likely. A retained placenta would usually manifest as large blood clots with lochia and would not cause a boggy fundus.

73. C) Hard, reddened mass

Mastitis is a breast infection most commonly seen in primigravidae and nursing patients. Symptoms usually appear between 4 and 6 weeks postpartum and include fever, chills, localized tenderness, and a palpable, hard, reddened mass. Blurred vision is a symptom of preeclampsia, and calf tenderness suggests deep vein thrombosis.

74. C) Use of assisted reproductive therapy

The use of assisted reproductive therapy (ART) has increased the occurrence of multifetal pregnancies. Approximately 25% of pregnancies conceived with ART are multifetal. Diabetes does not increase the likelihood of multifetal pregnancy. The likelihood of multifetal pregnancy increases with age and is not associated with younger maternal age at conception.

75. C) 500

For each 20 mL of breast milk produced, the patient must consume an additional 30 calories. This results in a dietary intake of an additional 500 to 1,000 calories each day in order to maintain patient weight. For breastfeeding patients, 200 to 300 additional calories are inadequate.

76. B) Umbilical artery
Umbilical arterial gas provides the most accurate information for determining neonatal acid–base balance at birth. It is a common standard of care to draw a sample from both an umbilical artery and a vein and compare the two samples to ensure that an *arterial* sample was obtained. The placenta lacunae, or intervillous space, is the maternal side where the nutrient exchange takes place.

77. A) Cerebral palsy
Magnesium sulfate given to patients at risk for imminent preterm delivery between 24 and 34 weeks' gestation has been shown to decrease the risk of cerebral palsy in those infants born preterm. Magnesium sulfate is given as a 4-g bolus followed by up to 24 hours of a 1- to 2-g maintenance dose. The drug is also used for patients who have high blood pressure or preeclampsia to decrease their risk for seizures, but this patient is normotensive, so seizures are not a concern.

78. A) Cord compression
Variable decelerations are a sign of cord compression, which can occur in the presence of oligohydramnios (amniotic fluid index of less than 5). Head compression may be seen as early decelerations on the fetal monitor as labor progresses and fetal descent occurs. Placental issues may cause late decelerations and may become an urgent matter.

79. C) Two amnions, two chorions, and two placentas
Dizygotic twins result from two mature ova being fertilized. This means that there will be two amnions, two chorions, and two placentas (although they may fuse into one). Monozygotic twins develop from one fertilized ovum. Most commonly seen are two amnions, one chorion, and one placenta. However, later division of the ovum will result in one amnion, one chorion, and one placenta.

80. C) Health Insurance Portability and Accountability Act (HIPAA)
The nurse has violated HIPAA. No healthcare worker should look at a patient's chart unless it is pertinent to the care of the patient. TheAffordable Care Act (ACA) regulates insurance coverage. The Administrative Simplification Compliance Act (ASCA) prohibits payment for services or supplies that a provider did not bill to Medicare electronically.

81. B) Fetal blood in maternal circulation
The Kleihauer-Betke test is a blood smear that can assess whether there is fetal blood in maternal circulation. It is usually done after injury or trauma to the abdomen to assess for fetal hemorrhage, which can be associated with adverse outcomes. If the test is positive, it is an indication that, if the patient is Rh negative, they should receive an Rh immunoglobulin (RhoGAM) shot to prevent isoimmunization in the next pregnancy. A total bilirubin lab value drawn on a newborn will assess the amount of bilirubin in the fetal circulation. A direct Coombs test assesses whether there are antibodies in the newborn's circulation.

82. A) Assess the patient's deep tendon reflexes
The patient presents with severe preeclampsia symptoms and requires magnesium sulfate to prevent maternal seizures. Before starting magnesium sulfate, the nurse must obtain baseline deep tendon reflexes (DTRs) and document the findings. A symptom of magnesium toxicity is depressed or absent

DTRs. Assessing the fundal height and obtaining the patient's weight are not priorities for patients with severe preeclampsia.

83. **C) Uteroplacental insufficiency**
Late decelerations are most commonly an indication of uteroplacental insufficiency. Fetal head compression is most commonly reflected on the electronic fetal monitoring strip as early decelerations. Umbilical cord compression is most commonly reflected on the electronic fetal monitoring strip as variable decelerations.

84. **B) Strongly predicts fetal acid–base balance**
When all of the fetal heart rate (FHR) components are normal on the electronic fetal monitoring (EFM), the tracing meets the criteria for a category 1 tracing. Category 1 indicates the *absence* of fetal metabolic acidemia and ongoing hypoxic injury. In other words, a category 1 EFM tracing is reassuring of fetal well-being and does not require interventions other than routine care. Fetal metabolic acidemia is anticipated with a category 3 tracing and requires immediate intrauterine resuscitation interventions or delivery to prevent further fetal hypoxia and fetal death.

85. **C) Nonmaleficence**
The provider is violating the ethical principle of nonmaleficence, which is the duty to do no harm and cause no pain. Although the patient initially declined an epidural, the provider is now knowingly ignoring requests for relief. Autonomy refers to the patient's ethical right to make their own care choices; administering an epidural despite the patient's refusal would violate autonomy. Justice refers to the application of fairness and impartiality in care; although the provider's action is unethical, there is no evidence that it is influenced by bias.

86. **C) Use of a birthing ball**
The use of a birthing ball is an example of a cutaneous measure to help manage pain during labor. Continuous labor support and music therapy are cognitive processes for managing labor that rely on auditory or visual stimulation to modulate pain.

87. **B) Intravenous ephedrine (Corphedra)**
This patient is experiencing hypotension, a common side effect of epidural pain management. Maternal hypotension can cause fetal distress and can lead to fetal hypoxia because the placenta is not being perfused adequately. Intravenous ephedrine (Corphedra) will help to quickly increase maternal blood pressure, helping to decrease fetal distress. Administration of 10 L of oxygen via nonrebreather face mask will not help treat maternal hypotension, and although it is part of intrauterine resuscitation, it is not the best choice for this patient. Intravenous ondansetron (Zofran) will help treat nausea, which in this case is a symptom of maternal hypotension; however, it will not correct hypotension.

88. **A) Baseline FHR of 165 bpm with increased accelerations and absent variability**
A baseline fetal heart rate (FHR) of 165 bpm with absent variability and increased accelerations is cause for concern because it could indicate fetal distress. Until fetal development has reached 32 weeks' gestation, preterm FHR characteristics include baseline heart rate of 155 to 160 bpm (compared with the normal range of 110 to 160 bpm), minimal to moderate variability, and accelerations of 10 beats

above baseline for 10 seconds. These characteristics are the result of an immature nervous system. The baseline goes down as the gestational age goes up; the variability increases, and the number of accelerations increases, including their amplitude and duration.

89. **A) Inability to focus or concentrate**
    An inability to focus or concentrate is a sign that the patient in labor is not coping well with uterine contractions and needs additional support. Patients coping well with uterine contractions will demonstrate inward focus and will relax between contractions. They may also engage in rhythmic movement during contractions and/or use rhythmic, focused breathing or vocalizations as self-focus or soothing measures.

90. **C) Vacuum-assisted delivery**
    A vacuum-assisted vaginal delivery is the preferred procedure for this patient because the fetal head is low enough and birth should be expedited because fetal distress is evident. Cesarean delivery would be the next choice if the vacuum assist failed to deliver the fetus, but it is not a first-line choice for this patient. An episiotomy may be warranted but is not routinely done and would not be a first-line choice for this patient.

91. **A) Reactive**
    A nonstress test (NST) can be performed to assess fetal well-being starting at 28 weeks. The criterion for a reactive NST that predicts fetal well-being before 32 weeks' gestation is fetal heart rate accelerations that are at least 10 bpm over the fetal heart rate baseline, lasting for at least 10 seconds. Beginning at 32 weeks' gestation, the criterion for a reactive NST becomes 15 bpm over fetal heart rate baseline, lasting for at least 15 seconds.

92. **B) Heart rate variability**
    Intermittent auscultation (IA) can be performed using a stethoscope, a DeLee-Hillis fetoscope, or a Pinard stethoscope, or it can be performed electronically using a Doppler ultrasound device. IA can provide the assessor with information on fetal heart rate, rhythm, and baseline, and it detects accelerations and decelerations in the fetal heart rate. EFM can also provide the assessor with fetal heart rate variability.

93. **C) Normal acid–base balance**
    The presence of FHR accelerations of 15 beats above baseline for a duration of 15 seconds is an indicator of a fetus with a normal acid–base balance and/or a normal umbilical cord blood gas pH of 7.19 or greater.

94. **A) "Delaying cord clamping for 30 to 60 seconds has several benefits for the preterm infant, including improved circulation and respiratory function and better blood flow to the brain."**
    Delayed cord clamping of 30 to 60 seconds is associated with significant benefits in preterm infants and should be done on all newborns delivered at less than 37 weeks' gestation. The associated benefits include improved transitional circulation, better establishment of red blood cell volume, decreased need for blood transfusion, and lower incidence of necrotizing enterocolitis or intraventricular hemorrhage. There is no evidence that extending the delay of cord clamping to 2 to 3 minutes is more bene-

ficial than 30 to 60 seconds. Additional time for the newborn to begin breathing on their own is not an associated benefit of delayed cord clamping.

95. **C) Continue to monitor**
The fetal monitoring strip shows early decelerations in the fetal heart rate, which can occur during normal labor in response to compression of the fetal head during contractions. No nursing intervention is required, although the nurse should continue to monitor. The nurse does not need to contact the provider or check the patient's cervix at this time.

96. **B) External cephalic version**
The nurse can expect the provider to perform an external cephalic version to help guide the fetus into a cephalic vertex position because the patient is not in active labor. A Cesarean delivery is not the best procedure to start with but can be considered if the external cephalic version fails. A forceps delivery is not indicated because the patient would have to be in labor and already 10 cm dilated to perform an operative vaginal delivery.

97. **B) Radial pulse**
It is essential to differentiate between the patient's heart rate and the fetal heart rate (FHR) by palpation of the patient's radial pulse while using a handheld Doppler device or an ultrasound device. Although it is important to monitor other patient vital signs, such as blood pressure and respirations, this is not the next step while performing IA for FHR assessment. The nurse must ensure that the heart rate they heard was fetal and not maternal to ensure fetal well-being.

98. **B) Placental abruption**
Placental abruption is characterized by a sudden onset of sharp, stabbing, mid epigastric pain that may or may not be accompanied by dark red vaginal bleeding. A placental abruption can be concealed or apparent, with increasing fundal height consistent with bleeding at the site of detachment. Cocaine use increases the risk for placental abruption. A patient with placenta previa presents with painless, bright red uterine bleeding that occurs during the second or third trimester without changes in the fundal height. Uterine rupture is characterized by sudden onset of abdominal pain and tenderness, vomiting, syncope, vaginal bleeding, tachycardia, or pallor with eventual hypotension and shock with fetal distress.

99. **C) Placental insufficiency**
An abnormal umbilical arterial waveform means that end-diastolic flow (AEDF) is absent, which indicates placental insufficiency. Fetal anemia would be assessed via Doppler ultrasonographic assessment of the peak velocity of systolic blood flow in the middle cerebral artery, not via an umbilical artery Doppler velocimetry assessment. Oligohydramnios may be a symptom of placental insufficiency, but it would be indicated by a low amniotic fluid index, not AEDF.

100. **A) Breech**
When, on cervical examination, the presenting part is a fetal foot, the fetus is in a breech position, where the head is near the fundus and the lower extremities are at the cervix. A cephalic position, the most common position near the end of a pregnancy, is when the fetal head is near the cervix and the

lower extremities are near the fundus. In a transverse position, the fetal lie is in a horizontal line in the maternal abdomen.

101. **A) Metabolic acidosis**
Metabolic acidemia is occurring when gases have a pH of less than 7.20, the partial pressure of carbon dioxide (PCO_2) is normal, and the base excess or base deficit is at least 12 mmol/L. Metabolic acidosis can result from prolonged or recurrent interruption of fetal oxygenation that has progressed to the stage of tissue hypoxia, anaerobic metabolism, and lactic acid production that exceeds buffering capability. A fetus with a prolapsed umbilical cord and grossly ruptured membranes, which were likely in that circumstance for the entire duration of a 2-hour car ride to the hospital, is presumably in this state of metabolic acidosis. Isolated respiratory acidemia occurs when the umbilical arterial gas pH is less than 7.20, the PCO_2 is elevated, and the base deficit is less than 12 mmol/L. This is typically related to brief umbilical cord compression—for example, during contractions in labor. Umbilical gas testing assesses for metabolic acidemia, respiratory acidemia, or a mix. With the absence of fetal respirations in utero, respiratory alkalosis would not be likely.

102. **B) Cesarean delivery**
The patient has a category 3 electronic fetal monitoring strip and has signs of a placental abruption. The best choice would be a Cesarean delivery because imminent delivery of the fetus is warranted. Cervical ripening would take too long to deliver the fetus because the patient's examination is remote from delivery. An intrauterine fetal blood transfusion would help with the fetal anemia, as a sinusoidal pattern is indicative of fetal anemia, but it would also take too long,. Thus, the best treatment would be to complete delivery.

103. **A) Epidural**
For patients with cardiac disease, an epidural is preferred because it provides excellent analgesia and avoids changes in heart rate and cardiac output requirements associated with pain and anxiety. Nitrous oxide would not provide adequate pain relief to decrease cardiac workload. A spinal block increases the risk of profound hypotension and should be avoided.

104. **C) "You should call your healthcare provider immediately. You may be experiencing very high blood pressure that will need to be treated."**
Significant maternal morbidity and mortality occur in the first few weeks postpartum. The nurse will identify the warning signs and educate the patient on the need to be evaluated as soon as possible for postpartum preeclampsia. Suggestions to drink water and get adequate rest are appropriate for someone experiencing postpartum stress but do not consider the signs and symptoms of postpartum preeclampsia. While postpartum preeclampsia can develop into a life-threatening emergency, the patient should be first instructed to call their provider. If the symptoms persist and the patient cannot contact their provider, they should go to the emergency department for evaluation.

105. **B) Cervical cerclage**
A stitch in or on the cervix is a cervical cerclage, usually placed at approximately 14 to 16 weeks in patients with a history of preterm delivery to help decrease the risk of subsequent preterm delivery. A B-Lynch suture is used to compress the uterus during a hemorrhage to decrease bleeding, and it would

not be seen on the cervix or while a patient is still pregnant. Infection would present as a friable cervix, with or without discharge and odor.

106. **C) 38°C (100.4°F)**
A puerperal infection should be suspected when a patient has an oral temperature higher than 38°C (100.4°F) on two occasions that are 6 hours apart during the first 10 days postpartum, exclusive of the first 24 hours. Temperatures of 37°C (98.6°F) and 37.5°C (99.5°F) are considered normal.

107. **C) Nifedipine (Procardia) and betamethasone (Celestone)**
Nifedipine (Procardia) as a short-term tocolytic and betamethasone (Celestone) for fetal lung maturity are indicated for a patient who is presenting in preterm labor, has no signs of infection, and can wait 24 hours to have the biophysical profile (BPP) repeated. The presence of oligohydramnios contraindicates the use of indomethacin. Magnesium sulfate may be used for neonatal neuroprotection, but the use of 17 α-hydroxyprogesterone caproate (Makena) is not indicated because it will not help prevent preterm delivery in the patient at this point.

108. **B) Lactogenesis II**
Lactogenesis II is defined as the onset of copious milk production that occurs 48 to 72 hours after birth when prolactin levels rise and progesterone levels fall. Lactogenesis I starts around midpregnancy and continues until 1 to 2 days postpartum, when prolactin levels rise and stimulate colostrum production. Mammogenesis occurs in two stages: during puberty and in the first half of pregnancy.

109. **A) Carboprost tromethamine (Hemabate)**
Carboprost tromethamine (Hemabate) should be avoided in a patient with a history of asthma. This medication is contraindicated because it can cause bronchospasm and bronchoconstriction, exacerbating respiratory distress. It is always important to review a patient's medical history and allergies before administering medication, especially in emergencies. Methylergonovine maleate (Methergine) should be avoided in patients with hypertension. Tranexamic acid (Lysteda) should be avoided in patients with a history of thromboembolic disorders.

110. **A) Duodenal atresia**
Polyhydramnios is defined as an excess of amniotic fluid with an amniotic fluid index (AFI) greater than 25 cm. Commonly known causes of polyhydramnios include duodenal atresia, blood incompatibilities/rhesus disease, infection, and diabetes. Potter's syndrome and intrauterine growth restriction are common causes of oligohydramnios, as are postterm pregnancy, diabetes, infection, and premature rupture of membranes.

111. **A) Initiate the massive transfusion protocol (MTP)**
Transfusion of blood products is integral to the comprehensive management of hemorrhagic shock in obstetrics patients. In the setting of an acute hemorrhage, massive transfusion therapy, an aggressive transfusion of blood products without lab results, is a vital part of resuscitation to reduce the risks of hemorrhagic shock and cardiovascular collapse. This protocol typically includes a set of the following: six units of packed red blood cells, six units of fresh-frozen plasma, one unit of platelets, and one unit of cryoprecipitate. The MTP would be initiated, and interventions such as a tamponade device, a Bakri

balloon, and other measures to save the uterus would be exhausted before performing a hysterectomy. This patient will likely need to be transferred to the ICU, but the priority is stabilization with MTP and stopping the bleeding.

112. A) 2.5
A cervix measuring less than 2.5 cm is considered to be below the 10th percentile of normal cervical length range and is associated with preterm labor and delivery. A cervical length of 3.5 cm or 4.5 cm is considered to be in the normal range and does not put the patient at an increased risk for preterm labor and delivery.

113. B) McRoberts maneuver
The McRoberts maneuver should be initiated immediately because the patient is showing signs of a shoulder dystocia, and this maneuver can help resolve a shoulder dystocia in up to 40% of cases. Gestational diabetes is a risk factor for shoulder dystocia because the condition increases the likelihood of fetal macrosomia, or being large for gestational age. An episiotomy is reserved for a shoulder dystocia that requires a manual extraction of the fetal posterior arm when there is not enough room for the provider to successfully perform the McRoberts maneuver. The Zavanelli maneuver is an intervention that consists of rotating and pushing the head back into the pelvis after all attempts to free the infant have failed.

114. B) Amnioreduction
The normal range of amnionic fluid index (AFI) is 5 to 24 cm. According to the ultrasound report, the AFI of the patient is abnormally high. Additionally, an enlarged skull is observed in the fetus, which signifies excess accumulation of amniotic fluid (hydramnios or polyhydramnios). This is treated by reducing the volume of amniotic fluid via amnioreduction. The desired amount of amniotic fluid is withdrawn using an 18- or 20-gauge needle with a larger syringe. Amnioinfusion may be indicated for conditions such as oligohydramnios, rather than polyhydramnios, where the volume of amnionic fluid is lower than the normal range. Amniotomy is conducted for the determination of thick meconium and the placement of an intrauterine pressure catheter or a scalp electrode.

115. A) Hydralazine (Apresoline)
The patient would benefit from blood pressure management with hydralazine (Apresoline) because the patient has a severe-range blood pressure, which can lead to more serious complications such as seizure or stroke. Magnesium sulfate is contraindicated because the patient has myasthenia gravis, and this medication can exacerbate muscle weakness. Labetalol (Trandate) is contraindicated in this patient because they have a history of asthma.

116. B) Magnesium sulfate
This patient is a good candidate for magnesium sulfate administration for neonatal neuroprotection. Giving magnesium sulfate to patients who present in preterm labor between the gestational ages of 24 and 34 weeks can lead to a decreased risk of cerebral palsy for the fetus. Gentamicin (Gentak) is not indicated because the patient has intact membranes and no sign of uterine infection. Misoprostol (Cytotec) is not indicated because the patient is preterm, so labor should be prolonged as long as possible for neonatal neuroprotection (in conjunction with corticosteroid administration) to help mature fetal lungs.

117. B) Preeclampsia

Preeclampsia is a potential complication of multiple pregnancy that can have consequences for the pregnant patient and the fetuses. Preeclampsia can lead to maternal eclamptic seizures and maternal cardiovascular disease. Congenital anomalies are potential complications that can affect the fetuses, but they do not affect the pregnant patient. Preterm delivery is a potential complication that can affect the neonates, but it does not cause maternal complications.

118. B) Place a gloved hand in the vagina to elevate the fetal head

The patient is experiencing umbilical cord compression due to cord prolapse, which is when the cord falls out of the vagina beneath the fetus and the fetus puts pressure on the cord, cutting off the fetal oxygen supply and causing prolonged bradycardia. This is considered an emergent situation and requires immediate intervention. The nurse will place a gloved hand into the vagina to hold the fetus off the cord. Repositioning the patient to their hands and knees is a suitable intervention to relieve the pressure on the cord, but it is not a priority. Once the fetal heart rate is stabilized, the patient should be prepared for delivery, typically via Cesarean section.

119. B) Flexion contractures of the extremities

Oligohydramnios is a condition in which the amniotic fluid volume is lower than predicted for the gestational age. Premature rupture of the amniotic membrane, along with the presence of oligohydramnios in the patient, can lead to orthopedic deformity such as flexion contractures of the extremities of the fetus. Anemia and hypoxemia are not associated with premature rupture of the amniotic membrane or oligohydramnios, but rather with placental abruption.

120. C) Manual reinsertion of the uterus

The patient is experiencing an inverted uterus, which can be life-threatening and requires immediate action to prevent postpartum hemorrhage. A manual reinsertion of the uterus would be the first-line procedure for the provider to perform because it can reduce bleeding and allow for the use of uterotonic medications, which will reduce the risk of recurrence of uterine inversion. A dilation and curettage would be performed to remove any retained placental membranes. Because the patient delivered an intact placenta, this procedure would not be necessary. A hysterectomy is the complete surgical removal of the uterus, which is not a first-line treatment in this situation.

121. C) Stimulation of the infant

Per the Neonatal Resuscitation Program (NRP), the standard newborn resuscitation algorithm uses airway, breathing, and circulation as a basis for stabilization of the newborn immediately after birth. The first step in this process for all newborns, including nonvigorous newborns with meconium-stained amniotic fluid, is to warm them, clear the airway, dry, and stimulate. Most newborns respond successfully to tactile stimulation and may not require additional interventions. Continuous positive airway pressure is not considered in the NRP newborn resuscitation algorithm until after labored breathing or persistent cyanosis is noted and the airway has been cleared. Endotracheal suctioning is not indicated, as the NRP recommends that resuscitation for infants with meconium-stained amniotic fluid should follow the same principles as for those with clear fluid.

122. B) Mature fetal lungs

Betamethasone (Celestone), given in two doses over 24 hours, is used to help mature fetal lungs and decrease the risk of respiratory distress syndrome in infants born prematurely by increasing fetal surfactant levels. Corticosteroids, such as betamethasone (Celestone), are also used to decrease inflammation, but that is not their primary use for this patient. Effort to prolong pregnancy in order to administer two doses of betamethasone (Celestone) to the patient and fetus is indicated in many preterm patients, but betamethasone (Celestone) itself does not prevent preterm birth.

123. B) Evaporation

Heat loss due to evaporation occurs as amniotic fluid on the skin is converted to a vapor; therefore, drying the newborn immediately after birth and removing wet blankets decreases evaporative losses. Conductive heat exchange occurs when two solid objects of different temperatures come in contact; examples include placing the newborn on a cold scale or a cold mattress. Interventions to limit conductive heat loss include providing skin-to-skin contact between the newborn and the patient. Radiant heat exchange occurs between solid objects that are not in contact. Interventions to limit radiant heat loss include using a radiant warmer after birth and moving the newborn's crib away from a cold window.

124. B) Greater patient mobility

The advantages of intermittent auscultation (IA) for fetal assessment during the intrapartum period include increased mobility for the patient in labor. In addition, IA can be used in conjunction with hydrotherapy and allows for a more natural labor and birth experience. IA can be used to assess fetal heart rate baseline, accelerations, and decelerations. Disadvantages include the need for increased staffing in the unit because IA requires 1:1 nursing care. IA also requires the patient to be low risk, does not have a printout to assess visually, and cannot determine fetal heart rate variability.

125. C) Hysterectomy

A placenta percreta occurs when the placenta grows through the uterus and attaches to other organs, most commonly the bladder. This can lead to life-threatening bleeding during delivery. If placenta percreta is found in the antenatal period, the most common practice is to schedule a Cesarean delivery in a hospital with the capability to handle high-risk situations. A hysterectomy is not always indicated for this complication, but if the bleeding is uncontrollable, it is generally an agreed-upon approach for most providers. A B-Lynch suture wraps around the uterus and compresses it to help control bleeding. It can be successfully performed for some placenta accretas, when the uterus is not attached to other organs, but it is less successful in placenta percreta. A Bakri balloon goes inside the uterus and inflates to compress the uterus in an effort to control bleeding. This would also be less successful than a hysterectomy in this dangerous situation.

126. C) Respiratory distress

Neonates born via Cesarean section do not undergo the mechanical compression of the chest that occurs during a vaginal delivery, and as a result, they may have increased fluid in the lungs after birth. The extra fluid in the lungs may increase the infant's risk of developing respiratory distress. Neither cold stress nor jaundice is associated with mode of delivery.

127. A) Corticosteroids
Corticosteroids should be given to patients with multifetal pregnancies between 24 and 34 weeks' gestation if the patient is likely to deliver within 7 days. Corticosteroids have been shown to decrease the incidence of neonatal death, respiratory distress syndrome, intraventricular hemorrhage, and necrotizing enterocolitis. Magnesium sulfate is used for neuroprotection in multifetal pregnancies when delivery is expected before 32 weeks' gestation because the greatest benefit is achieved at this time with the lowest risk to the patient and the fetuses. Tocolysis is recommended only for short-term use to allow time for corticosteroid administration or transfer to tertiary care because of the risks of long-term use.

128. B) Fetal scalp electrode
A fetal scalp electrode (FSE) should be offered to the patient at this time to obtain adequate tracing of the fetal heart rate and ensure that fetal distress is not present. An FSE would be able to successfully trace the fetal heart rate in any maternal position. An amnioinfusion is instillation of fluid into the uterus to help cushion the fetus and umbilical cord to decrease variable fetal heart rate declarations; it would not be effective for obtaining adequate tracing of the fetal heart rate. An intrauterine pressure catheter would be placed to get an accurate reading of uterine contractions, not fetal heart rate.

129. C) 85% to 95%
Healthy term newborns may take 10 minutes or longer to achieve a preductal SpO_2 above 95%. According to the Neonatal Resuscitation Program from the American Academy of Pediatrics, the term healthy newborn should reach a targeted SpO_2 range of 85% to 95% by 10 minutes of life. The range of 75% to 80% is the targeted SpO_2 range for a healthy newborn at 4 minutes of life. Similarly, 80% to 85% is the expected target range for a healthy newborn at 5 minutes of life.

130. C) Macrosomia
The fetus has macrosomia, which is defined as an estimated fetal weight above the 90th percentile, or an estimated fetal weight of 4,500 g or more. Hydrops fetalis can cause fetal edema, but the fetus having macrosomia does not in itself indicate hydrops fetalis. The pregnant patient may have hyperglycemia, which can contribute to macrosomia, but the fetus would have normal blood glucose levels or even hypoglycemia at birth.

131. C) Reactive
This nonstress test (NST) is considered to be reactive, which is defined as 20 minutes of a continuous fetal monitoring strip with at least two fetal heart rate accelerations of 15 bpm over the fetal heart baseline for 15 seconds after the gestational age of 32 weeks. *Nonreactive* refers to an NST that does not have at least two fetal heart rate accelerations on a continuous fetal monitoring strip in a 20-minute period. A positive test refers to a contraction stress test that shows fetal heart rate decelerations with contractions.

132. A) Forceps-assisted delivery
This labor complication is known as a head entrapment, which occurs during a breech delivery when the fetal body has been delivered and the fetal head is stuck. A forceps-assisted delivery can be useful in helping to deliver a fetus in this situation. A symphysiotomy procedure is an outdated procedure in which the pubis symphysis is cut to allow room for a vaginal delivery. It can lead to serious, long-term

pelvic problems in the patient. A vacuum-assisted delivery would not be helpful for this patient because the vacuum is applied to the fetal head, which is still inside the pelvis.

133. B) Episiotomy
The midline incision down the patient's perineum is known as an episiotomy. It is not routinely performed, but it can be used at the provider's discretion to help expedite delivery when there is fetal distress or a shoulder dystocia. It provides more room in the soft tissue and is cut from the vaginal opening to right above the anus. A cerclage is a cervical stitch that helps prevent preterm delivery in patients with a history of previous preterm birth. The Ritgen maneuver is used to help control the speed of delivery by gaining more control of the fetal head through applying upward pressure on the perineum with one hand while the other hand is on the fetal head.

134. C) Outlet
This type of forceps delivery is called an outlet forceps delivery because the fetal head is now near the perineum. Criteria for an outlet forceps delivery include the fetal head being near the perineum and the fetal scalp being visible at the introitus or the fetal skull having reached the pelvic floor. A low forceps delivery is when the leading point of the fetal skull is at +2 cm or greater and is not on the pelvic floor. A midforceps delivery is when the fetal station is above +2 cm, but the fetal head is engaged.

135. C) Magnesium sulfate
Magnesium sulfate should be ordered because the patient is showing signs of central nervous system excitability, which increases the risk for seizures. Magnesium sulfate decreases the risk of seizures in these patients. Ibuprofen (Motrin) is contraindicated in the third trimester of pregnancy and thus should not be given to this patient. Labetalol (Trandate) is not indicated because the patient's blood pressure is not in a severe range.

136. A) Category 1 auscultated FHR
Intermittent auscultation (IA) of fetal heart rate (FHR) is a two-tiered system adapted from the National Institute of Child Health and Human Development's (NICHD's) three-tiered system for electronic fetal monitoring (EFM). Category 1 auscultated FHR characteristics include an FHR baseline of 110 to 160 bpm, a regular rhythm, the presence or absence of increases from the FHR baseline, and an absence of decreases from the FHR baseline. An auscultated FHR in the category 1 tier reflects a fetus with an acid–base balance. Category 2 characteristics include those that are outside of category 1 parameters. Category 2 auscultated FHR indicates a need for further assessment, such as more frequent IA or application of the EFM to assess fetal well-being. There is no category 3 for auscultated FHR.

137. C) Terbutaline (Brethine)
The nurse can expect the provider to order terbutaline (Brethine) for this patient because they are experiencing tachysystole, or an abnormally high rate of uterine contractions. Tachysystole is defined as more than five uterine contractions in a 10-minute period. This abnormally high rate of uterine contractions can decrease fetal reserve and can lead to fetal distress and fetal heart rate decelerations. It requires an urgent intervention. Magnesium sulfate is used in labor to decrease the risk of seizure in preeclampsia patients, but it is not used to slow uterine contractions. Nifedipine (Procardia) can be used to slow uterine contractions, but the onset is slower than with terbutaline (Brethine), and it is not used for urgent situations.

138. B) To provide ongoing reassessment of the tracing

The tracing is category 2, fetal tachycardia, which is anticipated with maternal infection and/or fever. It does not require immediate intrauterine resuscitative measures or emergent delivery. This patient would require continued fetal surveillance, frequent reassessment, and management of the infection, and they would be allowed to continue their labor. An amnioinfusion would not be an appropriate order for this patient. The presence of fetal tachycardia alone does not indicate an urgent Cesarean delivery; the whole clinical picture must be considered. In this situation, the FHR baseline change is not directly related to fetal oxygenation status, but rather to the infection.

139. B) Reposition the patient to their side

It is important for the patient to avoid the supine position during labor because of the incidence of maternal hypotension and the impedance of uteroplacental blood flow. The nurse repositions the patient to their side to promote maternal-fetal exchange. Increasing oral fluids and starting intravenous fluids are not the first nursing interventions in response to hypotension but would be appropriate interventions if maternal position changes did not resolve the hypotension.

140. C) Nonstress test and amniotic fluid index

A modified biophysical profile (BPP) is used to assess fetal well-being and is comparable in outcomes to a regular BPP. The modified BPP consists of an ultrasound to assess for the amniotic fluid index and a nonstress test. Fetal breathing and fetal movement are two components of a regular BPP, not a modified BPP. Fetal kick counts are not part of either a BPP or a modified BPP.

141. B) Cigarette smoke contains toxins that directly affect the placental and fetal cells

Cigarette smoke contains many toxins that directly affect placental and fetal cell proliferation and differentiation and can explain increased risk of miscarriage. Active maternal smoking and passive smoke exposure have a damaging effect in all trimesters of pregnancy, not just the first trimester.

142. B) "Antibiotics help reduce the infectious and gestational age–dependent neonatal complications."

Antibiotics are administered intravenously in premature rupture of membranes (PROM) to reduce infectious and gestational age–dependent neonatal infections. Antibiotic treatment significantly prolongs latency after membrane rupture and reduces chorioamnionitis and the frequency of newborn complications, including infection, need for oxygen or surfactant therapy, and intraventricular hemorrhage. Prophylactic antibiotics are administered to laboring patients who are positive for group B *Streptococcus*.

143. A) Cesarean section

A Cesarean section is indicated for this patient. Delivering a fetus with a face presentation, mentum posterior, can be dangerous because it will hyperextend the fetal head and neck, causing complications such as cervical cord injury. Patients who are preterm have a higher risk for fetal malposition, such as a face presentation. A manual rotation to a vertex presentation is not indicated because it can cause further hyperextension to the fetal neck. A vacuum extraction is not recommended for patients who are less than 34 weeks' gestation and is not indicated with a face presentation.

144. A) Furosemide (Lasix) and lisinopril (Prinivil)
The patient is exhibiting signs of peripartum cardiomyopathy. Peripartum cardiomyopathy can develop as early as the third trimester of pregnancy and up to 6 months postpartum. It is diagnosed by an echocardiogram that will show a low ejection fraction and diminished functioning of the heart, or heart failure. This condition is up to three times more common in Black patients. Another risk factor is multifetal pregnancy. Symptoms include fatigue; palpitations; nocturia; shortness of breath, particularly when lying flat; lower extremity edema; and low blood pressure. First-line treatment in postpartum patients includes angiotensin-converting enzyme (ACE) inhibitors, diuretics, and anticoagulants, so furosemide (Lasix) and lisinopril (Prinivil) are the best medication choices for this patient. Magnesium sulfate and labetalol (Trandate) would be the treatment of choice if the patient had preeclampsia. A beta blocker would be first-line treatment if the patient were still pregnant. Nitroglycerin (Nitrostat) and warfarin (Coumadin) are not appropriate because nitroglycerin would further decrease the patient's blood pressure and is not first-line heart failure therapy. Warfarin (Coumadin) is an appropriate treatment along with an ACE inhibitor and a diuretic, but it is not the preferred medication when combined with nitroglycerin (Nitrostat).

145. B) Craniofacial abnormality
Exposure to cannabis, or marijuana, is associated with increased risk of intrauterine growth restriction, which can contribute to microcephaly or facial anomalies and smaller head circumference at birth. Chromosomal irregularity is associated with several factors, such as errors in the formation of gametes and exposure to teratogens, but there is no significant report of association between marijuana exposure and chromosomal abnormality in a fetus. Conjunctivitis is possible if the neonate is exposed to bacterial infection or chlamydia in the birth canal; it is not a risk of marijuana exposure.

146. B) Intravenous magnesium sulfate
Intravenous magnesium sulfate is indicated for fetal neurologic protection. When this medication is administered to a patient between 24 and 34 weeks' gestation who is at risk of delivering, it can decrease the fetus's risk of cerebral palsy. Intravaginal misoprostol (Cytotec) is not indicated because this patient does not appear to have any signs or symptoms of infection that would indicate the need to induce labor. Oral nifedipine (Procardia) can be used to slow labor down, but this patient is not in labor.

147. B) Fetal echocardiogram
A fetal echocardiogram would be ordered because this patient has several risk factors that put the fetuses at risk for cardiac anomalies, including type 1 diabetes, multiple-gestation pregnancy, and conception via in vitro fertilization (IVF). A biophysical profile is not indicated because the NST is reactive, which offers reassurance that the fetuses have adequate oxygenation at this time. An umbilical artery Doppler velocimetry assessment is not warranted because the fetuses have not demonstrated signs of distress.

148. B) A biophysical profile
The nurse can expect the provider to order a biophysical profile (BPP) because the nonstress test (NST) is nonreactive and fetal well-being needs further evaluation. Additional electronic fetal monitoring can

be ordered if the NST is nonreactive after 20 minutes, with a maximum of 40 minutes of a nonreactive continuous fetal monitoring strip before further evaluation is warranted. Since the maximum amount of recommended time has passed for the NST, additional electronic fetal monitoring would not be the best course of action. A BPP, which is indicated, will assess the amniotic fluid index, fetal movement, fetal breathing, fetal muscle tone, and fetal heart rate. A fetal echocardiogram would not be warranted with an NST because in-depth evaluation of the heart is not indicated.

149. C) Intrauterine pressure catheter

An intrauterine pressure catheter is a device placed into the uterus to detect uterine contractions when there is difficulty finding contractions with an external monitor. An amniotic hook is a device used to break the amniotic sac when the provider is rupturing the patient's membranes. A Bakri balloon is an internal device used to compress the uterus during a hemorrhage to control bleeding.

150. C) Prepare for immediate Cesarean section delivery

With complicated placenta previa, as evidenced by bleeding and a nonreassuring fetal heart rate, Cesarean section delivery should occur immediately, regardless of gestational age. Tocolytics may be initiated if bleeding occurs in conjunction with uterine contractions, but it is not the immediate action to be taken. The provider would not place the patient on bedrest because more urgent action is needed.

151. C) Cesarean section

The patient has signs of vasa previa, in which unprotected fetal blood vessels run through the amniotic sac and cross the cervix. The best course of action would be for the patient to be admitted for a Cesarean section because a vaginal delivery can be life-threatening for the fetus in this situation. If this condition is seen on an antenatal ultrasound, then a Cesarean section is planned in advance for the patient. Administration of corticosteroids would be appropriate if the vasa previa were diagnosed in advance because this condition can lead to preterm delivery, and often antenatal corticosteroids are given to the patient to help mature the fetal lungs. However, administration of corticosteroids at delivery could lead to adverse outcomes for the fetus. An amnioinfusion would be contraindicated because it needs to be administered via an intrauterine pressure catheter, which could cause additional damage to the fetal vessels.

152. A) Fetal scalp stimulation and vibroacoustic stimulation

Fetal heart rate (FHR) accelerations can be elicited spontaneously, through manual fetal scalp stimulation during a vaginal examination, or by vibroacoustic stimulation. The presence of FHR accelerations that are 15 beats above baseline for a duration of 15 seconds is an indication of a well-oxygenated fetus and is reassuring. Palpation of the maternal abdomen or repositioning of the pregnant patient may cause the fetus to change positions, but it is not a guaranteed method of inducing an acceleration.

153. B) External cephalic version

An external cephalic version is a reasonable intervention because the patient is not in labor and cannot be induced while the fetus is in a breech position. A Cesarean section may be necessary if the external cephalic version is unsuccessful, or if the patient had presented in labor and with the fetus in a breech position. An induction of labor is contraindicated in a patient whose fetus is in a breech presentation.

154. C) Metronidazole (Flagyl)
The patient has signs and symptoms of bacterial vaginosis (BV). The recommended treatment for pregnant patients with BV is metronidazole (Flagyl). Doxycycline (Vibramycin) is contraindicated in pregnant patients and would not be a first-line treatment for BV. Fluconazole (Diflucan) is used to treat yeast infections and is not indicated for this patient.

155. B) Placental insufficiency
Recurrent late decelerations are caused by placental insufficiency such as calcifications in placenta, hypertension in pregnancy, and abruption. Fetal baroreceptor response is seen with early decelerations caused by head compression and is indicative of a reassuring fetal response. Variable decelerations noted with fetal heart monitoring are most closely associated with umbilical cord compression.

156. A) Fetal fibronectin (FFN) swab
A fetal fibronectin (FFN) swab will help assess whether the patient is at risk for preterm delivery. A negative result indicates decreased risk for preterm delivery; a positive result indicates that the patient may go into labor within the next 2 weeks. The rupture of membranes (ROM) test is not indicated because this patient does not have any leaking of vaginal fluids. The group B *Streptococcus* (GBS) swab can be collected, but it is usually collected at 36 weeks' gestation, and any patient who presents in preterm labor will be prophylactically treated for the bacteria.

157. C) Rho(D) immune globulin (RhoGAM)
The patient is at risk for uteroplacental hemorrhage after being involved in a motor vehicle crash. Giving Rho(D) immune globulin (RhoGAM) will decrease the risk of isoimmunization. A blood transfusion is not indicated at this time because the patient is in the third trimester of pregnancy and hemoglobin and hematocrit are within normal range. Indomethacin (Indocin) is a nonsteroidal anti-inflammatory drug (NSAID) used to prolong pregnancy by decreasing uterine contractions. It is not indicated because the patient is not experiencing significant uterine contractions.

158. C) Educate the patient on the importance of staying until the social worker can assess the patient and provide adequate resources to take home
The nurse should show empathy and educate the patient on the importance of receiving the proper care prior to discharge. The referral process for patients who demonstrate risk factors for perinatal mood and anxiety disorders needs to be managed in an empowering, supportive way. Letting the patient know they are valued and that their concerns and feelings are important is a way for the nurse to give the patient the message that they deserve optimal care. Providing educational materials alone does not adequately evaluate the patient for postpartum depression. It is not appropriate to allow the patient to leave against medical advice without first educating them on the importance of the social work visit.

159. A) Amniotomy
Before internal fetal monitors can be placed, the patient must have rupture of membranes. The procedure of breaking a patient's water is called an *amniotomy*. An episiotomy, or incision down the patient's perineum, is not indicated for placement of internal fetal monitors. A hysterotomy, or transabdominal surgical incision made into the patient's uterus, is performed during Cesarean deliveries and is not indicated for placement of internal fetal monitors.

160. B) Respiratory acidemia
Respiratory acidemia occurs when fetal carbon dioxide (CO_2) cannot be easily diffused, causing increased fetal CO_2 levels. This can occur rapidly and also be rapidly resolved. Metabolic acidemia occurs when the metabolism changes to anaerobic, causing lactic acid levels to rise. Metabolic acidemia takes longer to develop and longer to correct. Due to the fetal circulation and the absence of fetal respirations, it is not likely that the infant experienced respiratory alkalosis.

161. C) Induction of labor
This patient is at term and has an unstable fetal lie. It would be most appropriate for the provider to order an induction of labor now, while the patient is known to have a cephalic vertex fetus. A Cesarean delivery is not indicated at this time because the fetus has successfully been flipped to a vertex position. An order to discharge the patient could lead to the patient returning to the hospital in labor with an engaged fetus in a breech position that would indicate the need for a Cesarean delivery in most hospital settings, so the best course would be to start an induction of labor now.

162. A) Placenta accreta
Placenta accreta is a type of morbidly adherent placenta, where the placenta has attached too deeply into the uterine wall but has not invaded the myometrium. Placenta increta is trophoblast invasion into the myometrium. Placenta percreta is invasion completely through the myometrium and into the surrounding pelvic structures, such as the bladder.

163. B) Complete blood count with platelets and complete metabolic profile
The nurse can expect the provider to order a complete blood count (CBC) with platelets and a complete metabolic profile (CMP) to assess for hemolysis, elevated liver enzymes, and low platelets because this patient has chronic hypertension with superimposed preeclampsia that may have progressed to HELLP (Hemolysis, Elevated Liver enzymes and Low Platelets) syndrome. Preeclampsia can affect both the liver and the kidneys, but blood urea nitrogen and CMP will not accurately diagnose HELLP syndrome. A protein-to-creatinine ratio is not indicated because the patient has symptoms of severe preeclampsia, which can be diagnosed without that test. Additionally, neither that test nor a CBC with platelets will help determine whether the patient has developed HELLP syndrome.

164. B) Intrauterine growth restriction
The fetus has intrauterine growth restriction, which is defined as a fetal weight below the 10th percentile. Hydrops fetalis is a condition that causes fetal edema, not growth restriction. Postmaturity syndrome may cause a fetus to stop growing, but it occurs after 40 weeks' gestation and is diagnosed after birth.

165. B) Leopold maneuver
The provider is performing the four-step Leopold maneuver, which is an external examination of the maternal abdomen to determine fetal lie. The first step is a fundal grip. A fundal height assessment would consist of the provider measuring the distance from the symphysis pubis to the fundus; it does not require a fundal grip. In manual palpation of a uterine contraction, the provider would not perform a fundal grip; instead, they would keep the hand placed between the fundus and the umbilicus during the duration of a uterine contraction to assess its strength and length.

166. **C) Small for gestational age**
Identifying patient risk factors is essential for identifying potential neonatal complications to prepare for interventions that can be provided to the newborn. Patient history of smoking, substance use, and low weight gain indicates a high probability of the fetus being small for gestational age. While many persons with substance use disorders may also drink alcohol, it cannot be assumed based on the patient information currently known. Newborn sepsis is not a potential complication of substance use disorders or low weight gain during pregnancy.

167. **A) Discontinuation of magnesium sulfate**
This patient is showing early signs of magnesium sulfate toxicity, so the nurse can expect an order to discontinue administration, along with a serum magnesium level to assess for the need for further interventions, such as administration of calcium gluconate (Gluconate). Furosemide (Lasix) by intravenous push would not be indicated because the patient is not experiencing signs of fluid overload, which is a side effect of preeclampsia. Intravenous hydralazine (Apresoline) is not indicated because this patient's blood pressure is not currently in the severe range.

168. **A) Emergency Cesarean section**
When the fetal head loses engagement in the maternal pelvis, it is a sign of uterine rupture. That, along with the uterine tachysystole and fetal distress, indicates that the patient requires an emergency Cesarean section. The Gaskin maneuver is a positioning technique used to reduce shoulder dystocia during labor; it is contraindicated in a uterine rupture because it can increase pressure on the lower uterine segment, potentially worsening the rupture. A vacuum extraction could be a viable option if a vaginal delivery were imminent, but this patient is only 7 cm dilated and is too remote from delivery to wait for the fetus to be born.

169. **B) Hypoglycemia**
Hypoglycemia (low levels of blood glucose) in the newborn occurs when the pregnant patient's blood sugars have been consistently high, causing the fetus to have a high level of insulin in utero. After delivery, the insulin level circulating in the newborn can remain high, but the newborn's blood sugar does not, because the infant is no longer receiving the patient's blood glucose. This causes neonatal hypoglycemia to occur. Infants born to patients with insulin-dependent gestational diabetes mellitus are often large for their gestational age rather than small; high glucose levels passed from the pregnant patient to the fetus result in fat development.

170. **A) "Have you experienced any epigastric pain?"**
The patient's headache and elevated blood pressure are potential signs and symptoms of preeclampsia. The nurse would assess for additional indications, such as visual symptoms and right upper quadrant pain or epigastric pain. Numbness in extremities is not a sign of preeclampsia. Itchiness of the skin can be a sign of cholestasis in pregnancy.

171. **A) Elevated fasting glucose**
The patient's symptoms suggest gestational diabetes that would be revealed by elevated fasting glucose. Gestational diabetes is a risk of all multifetal pregnancies. Elevated liver function tests would not

be suspected with normal blood pressure and no other symptoms of preeclampsia. Low hemoglobin would not be likely at this gestational age.

172. A) Intravenous antibiotics

This patient has signs and symptoms of chorioamnionitis and would benefit from intravenous antibiotics, such as ampicillin (Omnipen) and gentamicin (Gentak). Tocolytic agents are not indicated for this patient because they are contraindicated when there is evidence of uterine infection. Uterotonic agents are not indicated because this patient is in active labor at 6 cm dilation, 100% effacement.

173. B) Placental insufficiency

This asymmetrical growth pattern is typically associated with placental insufficiency. Aneuploidy (an extra or missing chromosome) and viral infection each produce a symmetrical pattern of delayed growth.

174. A) Low-lying placenta

Recent classification defines low-lying placenta as the edge of the placenta lying within 2 cm of the cervical os, but not covering it. With a partial placenta previa, the cervix is partly covered but not totally obstructed, compared with a true placenta previa, where the cervical os is completely covered. Placenta accreta refers to a type of morbidly adherent placenta, which has grown too deep into uterine tissue but has not invaded the myometrium.

175. A) Dilation

Dilation refers to how open the cervical os is upon assessment and is documented in centimeters: 0 cm being closed and 10 cm being fully dilated. Effacement refers to how thinned out the cervix is upon assessment and is documented in a percentage from very thick (0%) to completely thinned out (100%). Station refers to the fetal head's position in relation to the patient's pelvis and is documented as −3 (very high in the pelvis) to +3 (crowning).

9 ANSWERS TO POP QUIZ QUESTIONS

CHAPTER 2
POP QUIZ 2.1

The priority at this time is to ensure fetal well-being. The nurse should anticipate that the plan of care would include fetal monitoring, an ultrasound, and a biophysical profile. With no prenatal care and signs and symptoms of gestational diabetes, this fetus is at risk.

CHAPTER 3
POP QUIZ 3.1

Percutaneous umbilical cord blood sampling is an antenatal test that allows for direct examination of fetal blood cells. Other screening tests use fetal cells and material from the pregnant patient's blood or the amniotic fluid.

POP QUIZ 3.2

Variability is the most important predictor of fetal acid–base balance and adequate oxygenation when using electronic fetal monitoring. The presence of moderate variability indicates a fetus that is oxygenated and not experiencing acidosis at the time it is observed. Minimal, absent, or marked variability warrant further investigation and intervention.

POP QUIZ 3.3

The nurse would expect to use intrauterine pressure catheter (IUPC). The prior Cesarean section in this case puts the patient at greater risk of uterine rupture during labor augmentation. Due to the greater accuracy in measuring contraction intensity and resting tone with an IUPC versus palpation or external tocodynamometry (TOCO), this would be the better option.

CHAPTER 4
POP QUIZ 4.1

Cervical change is the definitive indication that a patient is in labor. Contractions, whether regular or irregular, do not truly indicate labor, nor does pain. The definition of labor is notable cervical change.

POP QUIZ 4.2

The most common side effect of regional anesthesia such as an epidural is hypotension. The nurse should cycle the blood pressure monitor every 3 to 5 minutes according to hospital policy. The patient should be supported in a tilted position, not lying flat on the back. The nurse should instruct the patient to report dizziness or nausea because patients may be symptomatic before a drop in blood pressure.

POP QUIZ 4.3

This patient has developed chorioamnionitis, demonstrated by fever and tachycardia. The patient's baby needs to be delivered promptly. Because dilation is still only 3 cm, the nurse should anticipate the need to prepare the patient for a Cesarean section and possible administration of antibiotics and antipyretics per physician order.

CHAPTER 5
POP QUIZ 5.1

The nurse should start taking vital signs (VS) at regular intervals, weigh patient pads to determine quantitative blood loss (QBL), and notify the provider immediately. Because the patient's fundus is firm, the source of the bleeding is likely a laceration of the cervix or vagina. The presence of bright red bleeding versus darker uterine blood is another clue. Repair of the laceration needs to occur as soon as possible to prevent further blood loss.

POP QUIZ 5.2

Endotracheal intubation should occur prior to providing positive pressure ventilation (PPV) to this newborn. From its appearance, diaphragmatic hernia should be suspected. Diaphragmatic hernia occurs when the diaphragm does not completely close during fetal development, allowing the bowel to enter the lung space. Lungs are not able to open fully to oxygenate the neonate. If the nurse gives PPV prior to endotracheal intubation, the pressure of the PPV may fill the bowel with air, which further compresses the lungs. The neonate will need surgery to correct the issue.

POP QUIZ 5.3

This newborn has imperforate anus. A fistula between the colon and either the vagina or the urethra allows the stool to pass. The newborn will need surgical intervention to repair the malformation.

POP QUIZ 5.4

Oxytocin release from the posterior pituitary initiates the letdown reflex. Oxytocin helps to contract the cells around the alveoli of the breast to release milk from milk ducts.

CHAPTER 6
POP QUIZ 6.1

Respect for patient autonomy applies to this case. The nurse may feel that the baby should be bathed immediately, but the patient has a right to delay bathing as long as the neonate is stable.

POP QUIZ 6.2

The principle of justice applies because the nurse helps to ensure that underserved patients receive adequate care.

POP QUIZ 6.3

The PDSA process (Plan, Do, Study, Act) can be used when implementing a QI project.

INDEX

abdomen, newborn, 108–109
abdominal assessment, 70
abruptio placentae, *144, 175*
accelerations, fetal heart rate, 58–59
acrocyanosis, 104
acute fatty liver of pregnancy (AFLP), 24–25
administrative liability, 132
AFLP. *See* acute fatty liver of pregnancy
17 α-hydroxyprogesterone caproate injection, *141, 173*
amniocentesis, 49–50
amnioinfusion, 67
amnioreduction, *160, 192*
amniotic fluid assessment, 41–43
amniotic fluid embolism, 85
amniotic fluid index, *197*
amniotomy, 74–75, *200*
ampicillin, *184*
anemia, 119–120
antenatal testing, 49–55
antiphospholipid syndrome (APS), 5–6
anus, newborn, 109
Apgar Score, 103
APS. *See* antiphospholipid syndrome
arrhythmia, 11
ART. *See* assisted reproductive therapy
assisted reproductive therapy (ART), *154, 185*
autonomy, 131

baby blues, 99
bacterial vaginosis, 31
Bakri balloon, *143, 175*
Ballantyne syndrome, *183*
bariatric surgery, pregnancy after, 25–26
behavior states, newborn, 110–111
benchmarking, *149, 181*
beneficence, 132
betamethasone, *147, 159, 178, 191*
biophysical profile (BPP), 53–54, *144, 175, 198–199*
birthing balls, 76, *156, 187*
Bishop score, 74
bottle feeding technique, 124
BPP. *See* biophysical profile
brachial plexus injury, 113–114
bradycardia, 56–57
breastfeeding, 122–124
breech position, *158, 189*
breech presentation, 83

carboprost tromethamine, *160, 191*
cardiomyopathy, 94
ceftriaxone, *145, 177*
cephalohematomas, *153, 184*
cerclage placement, *151, 183*
cerebral palsy, *154, 186*
certification requirements, 1
cervical cerclage, *159, 190*
cesarean delivery, 80–81, *144, 146, 148, 152, 158, 175, 178, 179, 183, 190, 197*
CHDS. *See* congenital heart defects
chest, newborn, 108
chlamydia infections, 32–33
cholelithiasis, 22
cholestasis, 23
chorioamnionitis, 87, *184*
chronic hypertension, 12
cigarette smoke, *197*
civil liability, 132
clindamycin, *148, 179*
coaching, labor, 76
complete blood count (CBC), *201*
complete metabolic profile (CMP), *201*
congenital heart defects (CHDS), 9–10
congenital heart disease, *147, 178*
contractions, *147, 179*
contraction stress test (CST), 50–51, *150, 181–182*
Cook balloon, 74
cord compression, *154, 186*
corticosteroids, *147, 163, 178, 195*
COVID-19, 32
craniofacial abnormality, *198*
criminal liability, 132
CST. *See* contraction stress test

data collection methods, 138
decelerations, fetal heart rate, 59–62
deep tendon reflexes (DTRs), *155, 186–187*
deep vein thrombosis (DVT), 30, 97
  compression stockings for, *146, 178*
diabetes mellitus (DM)
  gestational, 16–17
  medications for, 43–44
  pregestational, 16–17
  type 1, 18–19
  type 2, 19–20

Page entries that appear in italics refer to content in the practice test and practice test answer chapters.

DIC. *See* disseminated intravascular coagulation
dilation, *203*
dinoprostone, labor induction, 76, 88
disseminated intravascular coagulation (DIC), 27–28
dizygotic twins, *155*, *186*
Doppler ultrasound transducer, *143*, *174–175*
duodenal atresia, *160*, *191*
DVT. *See* deep vein thrombosis
dysrhythmia, 56

eclampsia, 14–15
electronic fetal monitoring, 55
endocrine disorders, 16–21
ephedrine, *156*, *187*
epidural anesthesia, labor, 78
episiotomy, 81–82, *164*, *196*
ethical issues, 131–132
evaporation, *162*, *194*
external cephalic version, 83–84, *157*, *189*, *199*
eyes, newborn, 107

fatty liver, 24–25
fetal acid–base balance, *155*, *187*
fetal assessment
　antenatal testing, 49–55
　heart rate assessment, 55–67
fetal echocardiogram, *198*
fetal fibronectin (FFN) swab, *200*
fetal growth evaluation, 51
fetal heart rate (FHR), *164*, *196*
fetal scalp electrode (FSE), 64, *163*, *195*
Foley catheter, 74
forceps-assisted delivery, *163*, *195*
formula feeding, 124
FSE. *See* fetal scalp electrode
fundal height, 92
furosemide, *198*

Gaskin maneuver, *202*
GDM. *See* gestational diabetes mellitus
general anesthesia, labor, 79
genitalia, newborn, 109
gentamicin, *148*, *179*, *184*

gestational diabetes mellitus (GDM), 16–17, *202*
gestational hypertension, 12–14
glucose tolerance test (GTT), 54–55
gonorrhea, 33–34
group B *Streptococcus* (GBS), 34

head and neck, newborn, 105–106
Health Insurance Portability and Accountability Act (HIPAA), *155*, *186*
heart rate assessment, fetal, 55–67
heart valve defects, 10–11
HELLP syndrome. *See* hemolysis, elevated liver enzymes and low platelets syndrome
hematoma, 94–95
hematopoetic anemia, 26–31
hemolysis, elevated liver enzymes and low platelets (HELLP) syndrome, 13–14
hemolytic disease, 28–29
hemorrhage cart, 135
herpes simplex virus (HSV) infection, 34–35
HIPAA. *See* Health Insurance Portability and Accountability Act
HIV infection, 35–36
human papillomavirus (HPV) infection, 36
hydralazine, *161*, *192*
hydrotherapy, 77, *148*, *180*
hypertensive disorders, 12–16
hypertensive emergency, 15–16
hyperthyroidism, 21
hypertonic uterine contractions, 64–65
hypoglycemia, 114–115, *202*
hypothyroidism, 20
hypotonic uterine contractions, 65
hysterectomy, *162*, *194*

IA. *See* intermittent auscultation
incision assessment, 93
induction protocols, 136
infections
　newborn, 116–117
　postpartum, 95–96

influenza infections, 37
informed consent, 133
intermittent auscultation (IA), *156*, *162*, *188*, *194*
intrauterine amnioinfusion, *151*, *182*
intrauterine growth restriction, *201*
intrauterine pressure catheter, 65–66, *199*
intrauterine resuscitation, 66–67
inverted uterus, *161*, *193*

jaundice, 115–116
justice, 132

Kleihauer-Betke test, *155*, *186*

labetalol, *183–184*
labor and birth
　complications, 83–87
　induction, 73–76, 87–88, *201*
　nonpharmacologic methods, 76–77
　pharmacologic methods, 77–79
　physical assessment, 69–73
　physiology, 69
　procedures, 80–83
　shorter duration, *147*, *179*
　stages, 71–73
laceration, 95
lacerations, 114
lactogenesis, 122
lactogenesis II, *159*, *191*
late preterm infant, 111–113
legal issues, 132
Leopold maneuver, *201*
liability, 132
limbs, newborn, 107
lisinopril, *198*
literature review, 137
lochia, 92
low-lying placenta, *203*

macrosomia, *163*, *195*
magnesium sulfate, *161*, *164*, *183–184*, *192*, *196*
massive transfusion protocol (MTP), 135, *160*, *191–192*
mastitis, 123, *154*, *185*
maternal physiology, 69

mature fetal lungs, *162*, *194*
McRoberts maneuver, 84, *160*, *177*, *192*
mechanical labor induction, 75
membrane rupture, *141*, *173*
　preterm, *143*, *175*
membrane stripping, 75
mental health, 99–101
metabolic acidosis, *158*, *190*
methylergonovine maleate, *145*, *176–177*
metronidazole, *200*
milk production, 122
misoprostol, labor induction, 76, 88
Montevideo Units (MVUs), 66
mouth, newborn, 106–107
MTP. *See* massive transfusion protocol
multiple gestation, 40–41

narcotics, labor, 77–78, 88
NAS. *See* neonatal abstinence syndrome
National Certification Corporation (NCC), 1
negligence, 133, *150*, *182*
neonatal abstinence syndrome (NAS), 117–118
neonatal group B *Streptococcus* infection (GBS), *147*, *179*
neonatal hyperbilirubinemia, 115–116
neonatal resuscitation, 101–102
Neonatal Resuscitation Program (NRP), *193*
neonatal seizures, 110
newborn
　body system assessment, 104–111
　breastfeeding, 122–124
　care and safety, 125–126
　complications, 111–118
　initial assessment, 103–104
　laboratory evaluation, 118–121
　neonatal resuscitation, 101–102
nifedipine, *159*, *191*
nitrous oxide, labor, 78, 88
nonmaleficence, 132, *155*, *187*
nonstress test (NST), 51–52, *156*, *163*, *188*, *195*, *198–199*

nose, newborn, 107
NST. *See* nonstress test

obesity, 25
oligohydramnios, 41–42, *161*, *193*
operative vaginal delivery, 82–83
opioid analgesics, *153*, *184*
osmotic dilators, 75
outlet forceps delivery, *164*, *196*
oxygen pathway and interruptions, 70
oxytocin
　discontinuation, 142, *174*
　infusion, labor induction, 75, 87

pain assessment, 92–93
palpation, 65
paracervical block, *148*, *180*
parent-infant bonding, 124–125
Patwardhan maneuver, *141*, *173*
peanut balls, 76
percutaneous umbilical cord blood sampling, 52–53
perinatal loss, 125
perineal trauma, *153*, *185*
perineum, 91
peripartum cardiomyopathy (PPCM), 94, *142*, *174*, *198*
Pfannenstiel incision, *145*, *176*
placenta accreta, *201*
placenta accreta spectrum, *145*, *177*
placenta percreta, *162*, *194*
placenta previa, *144*, *149*, *175*, *181*, *184*
placental abruption, *158*, *189*
placental insufficiency, *158*, *189*, *200*, *203*
polycythemia, 120–121
polyhydramnios, 42, *160*, *191*
postpartum anxiety, 100
postpartum assessments, 91–93
postpartum complications, medications for, 128–129
postpartum depression, 100
postpartum hemorrhage (PPH), 98–99, 135–136, *151*, *182*
postpartum psychosis, 100–101
postpartum recovery complications, 93–99

PPCM. *See* peripartum cardiomyopathy
PPH. *See* postpartum hemorrhage
preeclampsia, 14, *143*, *175*
pregestational diabetes mellitus, 16–17
pregestational hypertension, 12
pregnancy complications
　amniotic fluid assessment, 41–43
　antiphospholipid syndrome, 5–6
　cardiovascular system, 9–12
　endocrine disorders, 16–21
　gastrointestinal system, 22–26
　hematopoetic anemia, 26–31
　hypertensive disorders, 12–16
　infectious disease, 31–41
　rheumatoid arthritis (RA), 7–8
　Rh incompatibility, 5
　scleroderma, 8–9
　systematic lupus erythematosus (SLE), 6–7
pregnancy loss, 5
premature rupture of membranes, 86
preterm delivery, *144*, *175*
professional practice
　issues, 131–133
　perinatal core measures, 133–134
　quality improvement, 134–138
prolapsed umbilical cord, 85–86
prolonged pregnancy, 83
prolonged rupture of membranes, 86–87
prostaglandins, labor induction, 76
pudendal block, *148*, *180*
pulmonary embolism, 30, *146*, *178*

quad screen test, 53
qualitative research methods, 137
quantitative studies, 137

regional anesthesia, labor, 78–79
relaxation and guided imagery, 77
reliability, 138
research types, 137–138
respiratory acidemia, *201*
respiratory distress, *162*, *194*
retained products, 96–97

rheumatoid arthritis (RA), 7–8
Rh incompatibility, 5, 118–119
Rho(D) immune globulin (RhoGAM), 200
rhythm disorders, 11–12
Rutherford incision, *176*

scleroderma, 8–9
scoring, 2
severe hypertension, 136
shoulder dystocia, 84–85, *183*
sickle cell anemia, 28–29
skin, newborn, 104–105
SLE. *See* systematic lupus erythematosus
spinal anesthesia, labor, 78
spinal block, *148, 180*
statute of limitations, 132
stroke, 6
sudden unexpected postnatal collapse (SUPC), 104
suprapubic pressure, 84
syphilis, 38–39

systematic lupus erythematosus (SLE), 6–7

tachycardia, 56
thalassemia, 28–29
thrombocytopenia, 29–30, 121
thrombophilia, 30–31
tocodynamometer, *175*
tocodynamometry (TOCO), 65
tocolytics, 67
Trial of labor after Cesarean (TOLAC), 81

umbilical artery, *154, 186*
umbilical cord
  compression, *161, 193*
  entanglement, *142, 174*
urinary tract infection (UTI), 39
ursodiol (Actigall), *150, 181*
uterine activity, *148, 179*
uterine activity assessment, FHR, 64–66
uterine atony, *151, 153, 182, 185*

uterine rupture, *141, 173*
uteroplacental insufficiency, *155, 187*
uteroplacental physiology, 69
UTI. *See* urinary tract infection

vacuum-assisted delivery, *153, 156, 184, 188*
vaginal assessment, 71
vaginal birth after cesarean (VBAC), 81
validity, 138
variability, fetal heart rate, 57–58
vasa previa, *199*
vascular thrombosis, 5
VBAC. *See* vaginal birth after cesarean
vibroacoustic stimulation, *199*

Woods corkscrew maneuver, *145, 177*
wound vacuums, 93

Zika virus infections, 37–38